PRAISE FOR

If You'd Only Listen: A Medical Memoir of Gaslighting, Grit & Grace

"The book is an adventure story, tracking the travails and eventual successes of a liver transplant patient from the perspective of the patient's wife and caregiver. It is all true while at the same time reading like a medical thriller. I don't know how the author survived all these harrowing events and kept her sanity and sense of humor. She's one tough cookie."

>   —Robert A Nozik, M.D., Professor Emeritus,
>   University of California, San Francisco

"Highest praise for the author's compelling medical drama, *If You'd Only Listen: A Medical Memoir of Gaslighting, Grit & Grace*. She shares a cautionary tale of love and advocacy through her eyes as a life partner whose sweetheart is undergoing a liver transplant. Her strengths of compassion, brilliance and humor fortify her and shine through as she describes the experience of being vulnerable and mortal amidst the unpredictable course of major surgery and rehabilitation. Her skilled and colorful prose transports you into the immediacy of this frightening odyssey. I recommend this book for patients, family members and professionals involved in healthcare today. The Addendum is especially helpful."

>   —Susan Bartlett, LCSW, CCM, CBIS

"The phrase 'Do No Harm,' has been attributed to Hippocrates, 4th Century BCE. In 2001, the book *To Err is Human: Building a Safer Health System* was published by the Institute of Medicine, USA. For the first time, errors in the medical health system were dealt with, stating that the problem is not bad people in healthcare, but good people working in a system that needs to be made safer to avoid preventable medical errors. As the author painfully discovered and demonstrates in her book, sadly, this goal has not yet been accomplished."

−Benedicte Dahlerup, M.D., Neurosurgeon, Denmark

"The author's work is both gripping and instructional, a hard feat for any author. But it's also a warning. Sorenson writes not from the viewpoint of a doctor or a patient, but from the mostly unheard viewpoint of the loved one suddenly forced to single handedly take on the healthcare system in matters of life and death. She has turned her horrific experience with medical error into a fine literary account of the ordeal."

−Jonathan Odell, Author of *The Healing* and
Miss Hazel and the Rosa Parks League

"*If You'd Only Listen* is a finely written cautionary tale. A red alert for facing life-saving surgery−our own or that of a loved one. The author's intensity and humor make it a surprisingly delightful read. The love and caring are inspiring. The information about medical error at the end as well as recommendations for mitigation are invaluable."

−Carolyn Ingram, EdD, PCC, Psychologist and Coach
Author of *The Not-So-Scary Breast Cancer Book: Two Sisters' Guide from Discovery to Recovery*, with Leslie Gebhart, M.A.

"The author has spared no one, not even herself, in this engaging saga of saving her husband's life from hospital medical errors associated with his liver transplant. When it became clear that he could die as a result, she had to push through her midwestern Nice Girl conditioning to fight aggressively for him. Her husband eventually made an excellent recovery, but the author paid a steep physical and emotional price. She is determined to save others from a similar fate. In the Addendum, she discusses research on medical errors in the U.S. as well as recommendations for readers about how to prevent mistakes from ending the life of someone they love. Her information was very helpful to me personally when my husband needed surgery."

–Deborah Joy, PhD, Counseling Psychologist

"Despite the difficulties she went through, it's easy to be on this journey with the author. Her story of her struggle to save her husband's life after his liver transplant is personal and heartfelt, with the pacing of a medical thriller. Reading her work is like reading the work of a friend, along with resources at the end of the book for readers who may one day need to advocate for their loved one.

–Brooke Warner, Founder and CEO of She Writes Press and author of *Green Light Your Book*

IF YOU'D ONLY LISTEN

---◈---

A Medical Memoir of
Gaslighting, Grit & Grace

IF YOU'D ONLY LISTEN

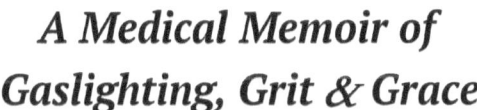

A Medical Memoir of Gaslighting, Grit & Grace

Rosie Sorenson, MA, MFT

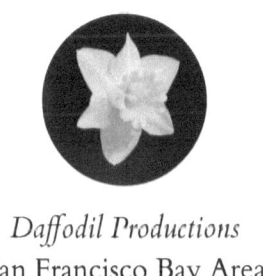

Daffodil Productions
San Francisco Bay Area

Daffodil Productions
San Francisco Bay Area

For permission, please contact: RosieSorenson29@yahoo.com

Printed in the United States of America

To protect privacy, names have been changed, except for Rosie's family and her cats.

The Introduction to *If You'd Only Listen* was a finalist in the San Francisco Writers' Conference Writing Contest, 2023, and was published in their anthology, *What We've Believed*.

ISBN 978-8-218-442460-0

Readers are advised to seek out the advice of their own personal physician or other medical professional or attorney. The information in this book is not meant to replace their advice. The author and publisher do not accept responsibility for any claims of adverse effects individuals may claim, directly or indirectly, from the information contained in this book.

Daffodil Productions does not have control over or responsibility for any third-party websites referred to in this book. All internet addresses listed in this book were correct at the time of going to press. The author and publisher regret any inconvenience caused if addresses have changed or sites have ceased to exist, but can accept no responsibility for any such changes.

To Steve West
My Indestructible Sweetheart
Glad you lived!

To the donor and family who made it all possible.
Thank you, thank you, thank you!

Happiness in Five Words

"Do Something for Someone Else"

—Oprah

CONTENTS

PART TWO

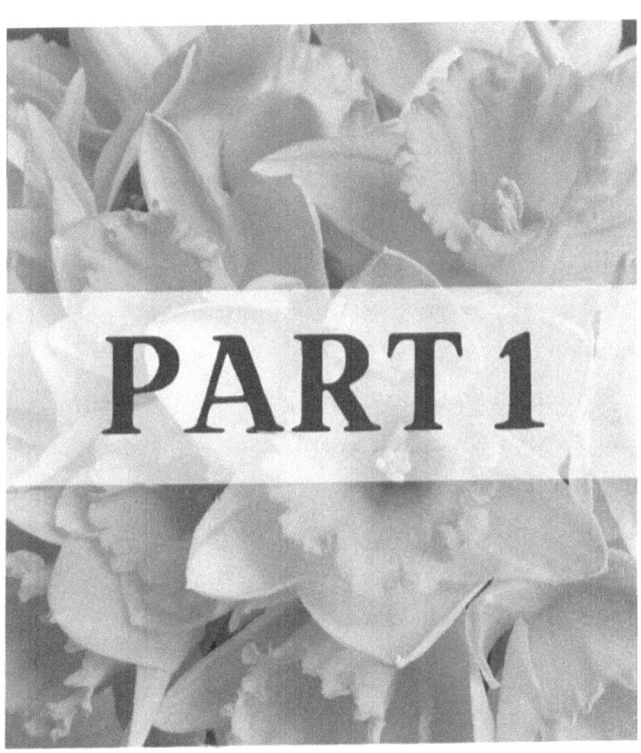

PART 1

AUTHOR'S NOTE

To write this story, I used my contemporaneous notes, emails and videos to document our struggles.

I've changed the names of every professional we encountered and have carefully avoided mentioning the name of the hospital or its location.

I've written this memoir so that others can learn from our frightening experiences and avoid them. What happened there can happen anywhere.

I have provided detailed information in the Addendum about the extent of medical errors in the United States and some recommendations about how to protect yourself and your loved ones.

I wish you good health and safe, effective medical care.

INTRODUCTION

It's 1:30 a.m. on Wednesday, March 17, 2015. I'm all alone in the cold cavernous hospital waiting room where I've shoved together three sizeable ottomans of hard burgundy vinyl, a makeshift place for me to lie down. Because they refuse to accommodate my 5'9" frame, I'm curled up in the manner of a cat, holding tight to my body heat, trying to halt my limbs' inexorable slide over the edge, like spaghetti slipping over the rim of a colander.

My carry on suitcase stands upright like a sentry. I had packed in a hurry—a crazy person tossing in a baggie filled with almond butter slathered on crackers, organic walnuts, a thermos of my favorite green tea, my cervical bed pillow, my phone charger, Steve's wallet, his medical ID necklace, who knows what else.

Steve, my soul mate of 16 years, is now lying on a steel table in the frigid operating room being prepped to receive a new liver. I'm calling upon every ounce of self control I possess to breathe smoothly—in and out, in and out—nothing to worry about, just in and out.

It's been four exhausting years since his diagnosis of non-alcoholic, cryptogenic, end-stage liver disease—a very long slog for him and for us as he slowly deteriorated and had to relinquish a teaching job he loved.

If you ever have a question about linguistics and the English language, Steve is your man.

Today is the day we've been waiting for, though not believing it would really come to this—the day his sick liver is being replaced by a newer, healthier model. Even though I know he's in the operating suite, nothing about it seems real. I'm playing possum with my feelings—fear and panic are not my friends. Steve and I grew up in the Midwest (Illinois, Indiana) where stoicism reigned and where sucking it up quietly was de rigueur.

After Steve's gastroenterologist informed him four years ago that he was suffering from end-stage liver disease and would eventually need a transplant, Steve said to me, "I felt a cold white wave of fear flashing up from my toes to my head, thinking I was going to die."

As the years of waiting dragged on and his physical deterioration continued, he retreated into a dispassionate turtle shell, leaving me to manage the logistics of our impending move to this out-of-state hospital, along with our unacknowledged roiling anxiety.

Now that the day has finally arrived, I confess to him how scared I am to let him out of my sight. He simply shakes his head, his brown eyes flashing, and says, "Let's just get'er done!"

Nothing more can I do but trail behind the two strong young men who wheel him into the surgical suite. My breath catches when the doors hiss shut, leaving me on the outside. Alone. Feeling icy and hollow, I weep as I traipse into the empty waiting room and find a seat, struggling to find my breath.

I've read that liver transplant surgery is considered an "ultra major" operation.

Are we strong enough to prevail? Or will I be bringing him home in a box? What if everything goes to hell? What then? I'm 2,000 miles from home. I've never felt more alone.

The only advantage of having had an abusive father is that in order to survive, I had to toughen up. I lived in a neighborhood full of boys, including my older brother, where I learned how to throw a punch with one hand and a spiral football with the other. And outrun them all.

But will I be able to rise above the vicissitudes of Steve's transplant? This has to work; it just has to.

There is no backup plan.

Steve barely escaped death during his evaluation week here at this same hospital two months ago. Due to the negligence of the evaluating gastroenterologist, who ignored my concerns about Steve's deteriorating condition, we ended up in the emergency room on our second day when the surgical resident on call nearly killed him by ordering a medication that could have ended Steve's life, just like that. Had I not been there and known that the med was dangerous for Steve and blocked the nurse from injecting him, he wouldn't even have lived long enough for a new liver. At least now he's getting a chance, but will it work?

And what if it doesn't?

★★★

Death, as an abstract concept, is easy to dismiss. *Nah, not me, not today.* But when Death shimmers around you, eager to claim someone you love, you can't breathe it away. You can't hum it away. You can only hold fast and hope Death moves on to someone else, not your sweetheart. Please, not your sweetheart; please, not your friend.

I don't know if I could have lived through the death three years ago of Carolyn, my funny best friend of 29 years, if not for two beloved kitties, Turtleman and Sonny Gray, who paved the way and whose deaths acquainted me with the architecture of grief.

This is how it begins: a squeezing, sickening tug in the gut that, if allowed to continue, will sink you to your knees. The only way to stop its progression is by taking deep, labored breaths. Your spine goes rigid, you're afraid to move. It can't be true. Maybe if you don't move it won't be true. Maybe if you stick to this spot right here it won't be true.

But then, somehow, the dreaded words sink in: "Turtleman's cancer has returned. Surgery won't help."

"Sonny Gray is old, his kidneys are failing."

"Carolyn died this morning."

The sharp intake of breath, the dizzy near-swoon, the tears, unattended by relief.

More tears, fought back at first. If you cry, it's real; if you don't, it's not. And later, the panic of nothingness that swoops in at 3:00 in the morning. You light a candle next to their photos. You say aloud how sorry you are, so very sorry, over and over and over again. You hope they hear you. You listen for a sign.

The fiercest element of grief is the void. No more cuddles with Turtleman during his treasured bedtime ritual.

Your home is now an empty pit of sorrow.

No more sweet greetings from Sonny Gray during my rounds at the homeless cat colony I care for. No more giving into his demands that I pet and talk with him before he will eat.

Losing them initiated me into the tribe of mourners, smacked me down in the ways of grief.

When Carolyn died, I was already familiar with the contours of heartache. I took solace from my furry boys whose passing taught me well.

As she lay dying, I sat at Carolyn's hospital bedside, holding her hand, telling my comatose friend how much I loved her. Her adult children and I consoled each other in the exchange of sweet and amusing stories about our dear Carolyn.

Later, at home, I lit a candle by her photo and took to my bed to read the Lee Child thriller I had just gotten for her. She'd think that was funny.

But just because you've been through Death more than once does not mean you're inoculated from its future ravages.

***

After I complained to our health plan coordinator in California about this near-fatal error and told him I was freaking out at the idea of bringing Steve back here for his transplant, he reminded me that the surgeons were excellent and that the patients they referred here had received good outcomes. He also informed me that our health plan had contracts with hospitals in two other states, and we were welcome to go visit them.

Neither of us could have survived that sort of schlep.

This has to work.

It's cold enough in here to preserve meat. I'm shivering under my black sweats and the pink fleece jacket I bought before we left California for this out of state hospital, thinking it would cheer me up. *Why do hospitals have to be so cold? To keep the germs drowsy,* is what I've heard, but who knows. More likely to save money. Hospitals have massive overhead to consider—must perform a lot of transplants to keep abreast of expenses. The combinations are staggering: liver & kidney; liver, kidney & pancreas; heart & lungs—miraculous pulsing bundles harvested from one generous gifter, to be flown here and installed into the welcoming viscera of a grateful recipient. We know nothing about Steve's donor—man, woman, where she lived, how he died, how many grieving family members did she leave behind, what had he planned to do with the years he thought he had left? We might never know.

A nurse, gowned in pale gray scrubs and hat, her mask dangling against her chest, had floated in on crepe-soled shoes to see me at 11:35 p.m. last night, to let me know that as Steve was being administered the happy drugs, he started spouting limericks. Perfect for St. Patrick's Day.

"Oh," I said, sitting up and reaching for my glasses. "I hope he didn't launch into his favorites."

"Yes, I'm afraid he did, but I know a few dirty ones, too, so we had a high old time." She laughed. I laughed. Just two gals in a bar, sharing a funny story.

That's my honey, I thought. Still talking. We've often joked about him being an out-loud linguist, one who loves nothing more than an overfull class of university students needing and sometimes wanting his wisdom about linguistics.

I often tease him, "You'll still be talking even after you're dead, won't you, Sweetheart?"

She also let me know that Steve's surgery had been delayed thanks to the opaque killer fog shrouding the airport. The private jet conveying his life-saving liver has been circling round and round for the past thirty minutes.

"What if there's an accident?" I said, my voice quavering. "How much longer before it can land and be taxied to us?"

"This happens all the time around here," she said. "We're in a fog belt. No need to worry."

Easy for her to say.

At 1:45 a.m., the nurse returns. No jokes this time. The liver has landed. Steve is doing well. I tell her that even though Steve is ill, he still possesses the natural constitution of an ox. All those years of childhood, working on the family farm in Indiana.

At 2:12 a.m., another nurse bustles out to tell me the surgeon has made "the cut." This is transplant speak for *we are slashing your husband from one side of his abdomen to the other.* My stomach clenches. The rubber is now meeting the road. It will be another seven long hours or more before we know if this has a happy ending. I think about the donor's family. There is no happy ending for them. How do you grok that someone has to die so someone else can live? If I were religious, I'd feel a chill.

"Are you okay?" the nurse asks.

"I'm really cold. Do you have any blankets?"

"Sure." She pivots and scurries down the hall as if she's off to save another life. She returns with four heavy covers.

Three TV's, one in each corner of the waiting room, are tuned to the "Wendy Williams" show. Blah blah blah blah, *Spanx*, blah blah, blah blah, *Botox*, blah blah blah. I search for the "off" button, but can find only the volume control. I reset it to low, but it's still too loud. My earplugs fail to keep the broadcast from laying claim to my mind, thwarting a craving to curl in upon myself, to shut out the babble. To dive down for one worry at a time, hauling it up to polish the rough edges like a gemstone until it's less likely to nick me and make me bleed.

Repeating the process seriatim, I struggle to make sense of the nonsensical.

Chapter One

WAITING, WAITING

H ow exactly did we end up here, far from home, Steve on the operating table surrounded by surgeons and nurses, me on the ottoman cluster, alone?

When he received his diagnosis of "non-alcoholic, cryptogenic, end-stage liver disease" in 2011 we were gobsmacked. How could this happen? He'd never been a drinker, never took drugs, didn't have Hep C, so how the fuck did this happen? His doctors couldn't determine the cause, but did tell us with certainty that he would eventually require a liver transplant. In our folie à deux, we felt confident that "eventually" would never come for Steve, that Steve would beat down this monster, keep it from stealing his precious liver. But, no. The monster won. Steve's deterioration progressed more slowly than a peach rotting in the sun, but nonetheless, it steadily advanced: the swollen legs and belly from fluid congestion (ascites); the petechiae (small red dots caused by bleeding into the skin, due to low platelets); the yellow sclera; the bouts of encephalopathy from the buildup of ammonia in the brain; the confusion relieved only by Xifaxan or Lactulose; the five hospitalizations for menacing infections and fatigue. The damn fatigue.

Because livers are scarce in our home state of California, thanks in part to helmet laws and a population of which only 40% are registered donors, his doctor recommended we travel to another state with no helmet laws, where our health plan had a contract with a hospital for transplants and where 55% of the population are registered donors.

Steve had been on the transplant waiting list near our home at the University of California, San Francisco, for four years and there were still 99 people ahead of him. Because of his worsening condition, we finally scheduled Steve for an evaluation at the new out-of-state hospital to examine Steve, review all his records and determine whether or not he is a good candidate for their program.

No time to waste.

Steve's belly had become so distended from ascites he looked fifteen months pregnant. Belts could no longer hold up his trousers. We selected a pair of rainbow suspenders, which were hell to manipulate whenever I had to escort him into the tiny lavatory on the four-hour United Airlines flight. Diuretics have a way of scolding the fluid right out of your body. And often. The flight attendants eyed us each time with suspicion. I waved them off, saying, "He needs my help," in the tone of someone who really means, *Don't mess with me. He's dying and I'm tired. And perhaps a bit cranky.* Fear has a way of tunneling your vision to a pinpoint so you can laser in on the most critical threats.

Steve's evaluation was to have been a four-day affair during which the transplant team of gastroenterologist, social worker and surgeons would examine him, review his previous medical records, conduct extensive testing and render a verdict.

An audition of sorts.

It was not supposed to be a tutorial on all the ways a patient can die in a hospital. As I would later find out, as many as 371,000 patients die every year in the U.S. from preventable medical errors.

A staggering, sobering sum.

Chapter Two

OFF TO MEET THE WIZARD

Sunday, January 11, 2015
11:30 p.m.

We arrive in this new city, home to the hospital where Steve will be evaluated for a liver transplant.

Exhausted from the flight and the taxi ride, we stumble into the old hotel. Everything about it is tired—the dun carpet, the lackluster paint, the jaundiced light fixtures. The elevator creaks us up to the fourth floor. It's as if the anguish of previous patients and families who have taken up quarters here has brought the hotel to its knees. It begs for young, frisky inhabitants to inject its halls with laughter, to exhale the stale air.

We step out of the elevator, sleuth the numbered plaques on the wall directing guests to their rooms. We turn left and five doors down pause at the first of our adjoining rooms—my fitful sleep requires a separate room to protect me from Steve's sonorous renderings.

I slip the key card into the first door and shove it open. Inside, the room looks as though it belongs to a different hotel. The laminate furniture gleams; the bedspread betrays no sense of wear,; the ivory drapes hang crisp and stalwart. Turquoise threads weaving throughout the brown tweed carpet spark some life. There's even a small refrigerator and a microwave.

"So far, so good," I say as Steve collapses into an overstuffed chair. He's about as spent as a human can be. I undo the lock on the adjoining door in my room, hustle out to the hall, nudge into his room and open it from his side.

The bellhop, an older man dressed in a black suit, white shirt and red bowtie, his Old Spice ascendant, knocks on my door and wheels the luggage cart into the room. I ask him to set mine near the closet and to wheel Steve's through the adjoining door and into his room. I hand him a tenner. We are tired and grateful.

"I'm gonna go get ready for bed," Steve says. At 6'2" and 230 pounds, much of the weight from ascites—unwanted fluid floating around in his body—he slowly pushes up from the chair and scuffs into his room.

"OK, Sweetie. I'll be there in a bit." I glance around at all that needs to be unpacked. I flop down on the bed. We've been upright for nineteen hours. Now maybe I can relax. The mattress is my new best friend.

I'm caught by a metallic rattling from Steve's room, punctuated by "Goddammit." I pop up and rush in to find him standing before the drapes, furiously yanking on the pull in his hand. "Goddammit." The curtain rod is angled downward, the full drape and its diaphanous lining now hang on a slant like a defiled prom dress.

"What the hell are you doing?" I say, trying but failing to be calm.

"I couldn't get this thing to close . . . . "

"Stop. Just stop." I swoop in to take the pull from his hand. I look up, assess the damage and, though tired and annoyed, I can't help but snicker. I fling out my left arm, Vanna White style, and say, "Well, Hon, you did this up proud. The staff's going to think you had a mad monkey in here. Or that we had us some hot, primitive sex." We can't stop laughing.

I hug him and say, "Well, fuck. Whaddya say we just leave it and go to bed?"

Monday, January 12, 2015
8:30 a.m.

No appointments scheduled for today. Steve sleeps in while I taxi to Whole Foods to lay in some provisions to supplement the cafeteria fare for the next few days.

I chalk up Steve's confusion of last night to the stress of the day—the schlepping of the luggage, the standing in lines, the frequent trips down the crowded aisle to the lavatory in the plane, the interminable flight, the harried taxi ride—we're done in. Xifaxan is supposed protect him from a rise in ammonia, which causes hepatic encephalopathy, but, worry upon worry, he's more confused now than he has been in months. Simple tasks elude him: the drape caper of last night; the removal of his suspenders, pants and pressure socks; the unpacking and organizing of his clothes and his toiletries. A sick liver simply can't filter out the bad stuff like it's supposed to.

A new liver can't come fast enough.

I return from Whole Foods to find him sitting on the edge of his bed, dressed, except for socks and shoes, watching a NASCAR race on TV. I hand over his espresso.

"Do you want me to warm that up?" I ask.

He shakes his head. "It's fine." He wants to know what the plan is for the next few days. I've explained the details of his upcoming evaluation schedule, multiple times, but I know the information does not land. A scrim floats on the watery curve of his eyes.

Reminds me of what I see whenever I try to convey something to our cat: "Please don't do that, Sugar, it hurts Mommy." I convince myself that if I speak slowly and clearly, she will get it.

Never happens.

This is the day we had hoped would never come. Our heads have been poised in a guillotine for the four years since his diagnosis. We'd adopted a mask of normality despite knowing the blade could plunge at any time. Prone to infections because of his failing liver, he'd had several close calls when he was hospitalized with septicemia. He rebounded each time, but whenever his temperature overshot 100.4°, I had to drive hell bent for leather to the emergency room. The fact that he could tolerate massive doses of powerful antibiotics for these and subsequent bouts of illness flooded me with gratitude. My honey was not going down without a fight.

To keep from flipping out, I have to tuck away the plain fact that my sweetie is nearly as fragile as a baby bird and that I'm responsible for keeping him alive until he receives his new liver.

I admire people who leap into parenthood, believing they are the best and only ones to keep a baby safe.

That sort of faith has never knocked on my door.

Tuesday, January 13, 2015
8:30 a.m.

Steve's appointments begin at 11:00 a.m.—first the blood draw, then a parade of meetings with the liver team members, a gauntlet of sorts. I wake up, shower, dress in my freshly pressed black pants, red suit jacket, ballet flats, friendly smile. Anything

I can do to impress upon the team that Steve deserves a liver and that I am competent to take care of him.

I dash downstairs to the cafeteria, corral some eggs and toast. Nothing else on the menu appeals: fried potatoes, greasy bacon. We're no longer in the land of Alice Waters and fresh California organic everything.

I return to the room, set my victuals on the desk, knock on the adjoining door and creep slowly into his room. "Rise and shine, Sweetheart, this is your big day!"

What if they don't accept him?

Steve rolls over, groggy, and says, "Huh?"

I sit down next to him, kiss his cheek. "Remember? You have your appointments today—about your liver."

"Oh, right," he says and sits up, slowly pivoting his fluid-laden tree-stump legs onto the floor and starts toward the bathroom. As soon as I hear the shower running, I return to my room to wolf down my breakfast. Steve prefers a vanilla Glucerna with his morning pills, saving real food for later.

After twenty minutes, I slip back into his room. No Steve. Cold fear lights me up. I rush to the bathroom to find him standing at the door-length mirror, wearing only his blue oxford shirt and underwear, no trousers, no socks, no shoes.

"What's going on, Honey?" I say, fear growing tight in my gut. His shirt is buttoned all cattywampus.

"I can't," he says in a halt while trying to manipulate the buttons. "I can't get this to work." My heart breaks. This man whom I've loved for sixteen years after we met at a Yoga retreat, the smartest man I know, cannot figure out how to button his shirt?

"Here, Steve, let me help you." I do a quick undo/redo. He shakes his head. He's still my beautiful brilliant Steve, but right now he moves more slowly than the Rain Man.

"Ok, now," I say. "Let's get your pants and shoes on. We don't want to be late." I take his hand and lead him to the bed.

We've gone through this before when he experienced episodes of confusion from an increasing buildup of ammonia in the brain. When the liver is damaged, its filtering capabilities are reduced, thus the increase of ammonia and brain fog.

He resists my help, but needs it. The day has barely begun and I want to cry. My whip-smart man with a Ph.D. from UCLA, fluent in Turkish and a few other languages, can hardly function now. He sits on the bed while I gather his trousers and pressure socks. They're meant to hug his legs in a tight embrace to keep the swelling in check but are monstrous to pull on, even with his special appliance. Forty minutes later, he's dressed and ready to leave.

I hail a cab and we arrive at the hospital with twenty minutes to spare. Steve shuffles slowly when he's having a bout of encephalopathy, at least I think that's what's happening now. I'm counting on the gastroenterologist to tell us.

Once the blood draw has been completed, we ride up the escalator to find the social worker's office. Mary, a short smiling brunette, is waiting for us. She asks her questions; we ask ours. I tell her about Steve's confusion, about his inability to button his shirt, that I'm concerned about his ammonia level. She says the GI doctor will handle that and hands us a packet of general information, but, as I am soon to find out, she has failed to provide the most critical detail of all—whom to call in case of an emergency while we're staying at the hotel.

We move on to the office of Dr. Yilmaz. I describe Steve's confusion to him, how it's gotten worse, how he couldn't button his shirt this morning, how I think that he needs an ammonia test and then some Lactulose, the sweet sticky liquid that draws ammonia out of the body, but the doctor is so impressed that Steve can converse with him in fluent Turkish that I've been disappeared. Steve may sound coherent at this moment, but I know him intimately, and what the doctor is hearing and seeing is not a normal Steve.

Dr. Yilmaz attends only to Steve, reverting to English to inform him that if he is accepted for a transplant and "listed," he can expect to move here and stay for up to six months while he awaits a liver. After he performs a brief exam, he sends us on our way to the financial counselor who reviews our insurance. Steve is scheduled to meet the surgeon on Thursday.

I am mired in regret that I did not press Dr. Yilmaz more firmly about an ammonia test, but these people had the power to say yay or nay to giving Steve a liver, so who was I to rock the boat so soon?

And who could have predicted that his oversight might have led to Steve's death.

Chapter Three

LET THE GAMES BEGIN

Tuesday, January 13, 2015
12:30 p.m.

B ack in our hotel, Steve naps while I slip down to the restaurant to gather some salads. I wake him to eat. The site of the drapes canted into a heap on the chair makes me laugh. "How much do you think this is gonna cost us?" I say. With Steve, nothing's too sacred to laugh about.

Once Steve drifts into sleep again, I hurry downstairs to the Business Center to use their computer to email friends and family. They're on edge and eager for news. I hustle back for an overdue nap, kick off my shoes and collapse onto the bed.

I'm wound tighter than a spool of mercerized thread, my mind treadling: *What if they don't accept him?* A death sentence, for sure. *What if they accept him but want him to stay now to wait for his liver?* I'll have to ask his son to fly in to watch over him while I pull together a plan at home for our absence. *Who will I get to take care of our two cats, one of whom needs asthma medication every other day? Who will sort our mail and pay our bills?* I'm fucking exhausted. So many ways for this to go sideways, and it's all down to me. No matter what, I must make this work. Ours is a mid-life romance, sixteen years and counting, and I'm determined to make it to twenty.

Wednesday, January 14, 2015
6:30 a.m.

Only one appointment today—an ultrasound of Steve's liver.

"What are we doing today?" he asks for the umpteenth time. If we were at home, if this liver business had never happened, we'd be engaging in our usual banter—debating the meaning of a particular word, racing to the dictionary to see who was right, collapsing on the bed in a haystack of laughter.

We're so hard core that we'd once engaged in a heated discussion about the diagramming of a sentence. In my day, a hush of reverence enveloped the diagramming of an English sentence. Why, if you could diagram, you could conquer the world! Whenever Mrs. Youngberg, my seventh grade English teacher, sought a volunteer to diagram a particular sentence on the blackboard, I would thrust up my hand and hustle to the front of the class. Grabbing the chalk, my hands a flurry of anticipation, I'd diagram the subject/predicate/noun/verb/adjective, just like that.

I am Diagrammer. Hear me roar!

In my bones, I knew that this was the right way to understand a sentence, so when Steve casually mentioned to me over lunch one day that those beloved Reed Kellogg diagrams were passé, that "they don't represent the language as it really is," I started thinking d-i-v-o-r-c-e.

"Them's fightin' words, Mister," I said.

"Syntactic trees," he continued in his most professorial tone, "are the only way to provide a visual representation of the underlying structure of a sentence." He sipped his Earl Grey.

"Balderdash!" I cried in churlish response and fiddled with my spoon. "What do your poor students think about this?" I asked, leaning back in my chair. Steve teaches linguistics in a TESOL (Teachers of English to Speakers of Other Languages) program in the Extension at the University of California, Berkeley.

"They get all nostalgic and defensive about the Old Way," he said and reached for a scone.

"Well, of course. They think they're special because they were the big dogs of diagramming in their day. But you come along with your fancy-pants syntactic trees and tell them that everything they have believed all their lives is wrong."

"That's right," he said.

"Can't you see how this undermines their entire world view? I mean, if they were wrong about diagramming, what else might they be wrong about? It's too much to bear."

We stared at each other across the kitchen table.

"They hate you, don't they?" I said.

"Afraid so."

"You know what you are? You're the Grammatical Antichrist!"

"Yes. But what they hate more than anything is that I have *fun* with this stuff."

"Well," I said, standing up and planting my hands on my hips, "on behalf of all your students, I feel compelled to say how 'bout you take your syntactic trees and shove 'em! We know what we know, and no one's going to take our sacred diagrams away from us, you hear?"

But instead of jousting about words at home, we're now several thousand miles away, hoping for a miracle. I want and need him to get his words back.

"We have to get you ready for your ultrasound, Steve. Can you hurry up a bit?" Of course he can't hurry up. I can only do so much because of my own physical limitations—the aftermath of a car accident several years ago and the subsequent surgeries that failed to deliver me from pain and fatigue and the onset of fibromyalgia. Where would I be without my ibuprofen?

My phone rings. "I'm going to get that while you get dressed," I say and shove off to my room. It's Jan, Steve's older sister from Maine.

"So far so good, I guess," I tell her, "but his confusion is much worse than it was at home. The Xifaxan is supposed to take care of all of this; so I don't know why he's having so much confusion."

I cave onto the bed.

"What do the doctors say?"

"Well, that's the thing. I explained it to the social worker and the gastroenterologist, and they brushed me off. Steve's having an ultrasound this morning, but after that, I'm going to call the social worker and see if we can get him tested." I don't want to alarm Jan more than necessary. *I'm here, I'm in control, I'll take good care of your brother.*

"Let me know what happens," she says. "I'm worried about him." Jan delights in telling everyone her favorite childhood story about the time she fainted when she heard her mother had given birth to yet another boy (Steve.) Her three brothers, one older, two younger, overwhelmed her. She was seven at the time and longed for a baby sister. To even the odds, Steve was supposed to have been a "Becky."

Jan's disappointment evaporated, though, one wintry morning on the farm in Indiana. As she tells it, there he was—little three-year-old Stevie, stuffed into his snowsuit, idling on a snowy hillock a few yards away.

For some reason, she'd suddenly whirled around, and when she saw Steve's angel face haloed in a sunbeam, her heart ignited with an overwhelming love for him that has never faltered.

"I know, Jan. I'll keep you posted. Love ya." I sigh and push off the bed.

I hustle into Steve's room. He's still sitting upright on the side of the bed, dressed in a shirt and trousers, but no socks, no shoes. He's staring at the floor.

"What's going on, Honey?" I say. "You need to put on your socks. We don't want to be late for your appointment." I sidle next to him.

"I can't," he says and reaches for his shoe.

"No, Sweetie, that's your shoe," I say. "Here, let me get your socks." We struggle for fifteen minutes to pull up his pressure stockings, just so. We slip on his loafers. I wrap him in a hug and kiss his cheek. "I'm going to take good care of you, Honey, don't worry."

I fear I'm not up to this, but I can't tell him that I'm already spent and it's only Wednesday.

I have to hold it together until Friday afternoon when we're scheduled to fly home. I'm placing a lot of trust in these people. Most health care providers I've known are dedicated and talented and take their Hippocratic Oath seriously, but that doesn't mean they don't screw up on occasion, as we are about to experience.

All physicians are bound by the oath of Hippocrates, the famous Greek physician of the fourth Century BCE who said, "I swear by Apollo the physician, and Aesculapius the surgeon, likewise Hygeia and Panacea, and call all the gods and goddesses to witness, that I will observe and keep this underwritten oath, to the utmost of my power and judgment."

The shorthand for his oath became: "First Do No Harm."

Perhaps an addendum should have been offered: "But if we screw up, please do accept our most sincere apologies."

Let us hope everyone at this hospital takes their oath seriously.

I jostle myself off the bed and stand in front of him, extending my hand. "OK, Sweetheart, you look fine. Let's go," I say. He rises. I slip my arm through his, snatch my day bag on the way out and together we slow-walk the hall to the elevator.

After the brief taxi ride, we arrive at the gleaming steel and glass hospital lobby. The strains of classical music echo off the high ceiling. I lead Steve over to the information desk where a kindly white-haired woman named Roberta awaits. "Can you please tell us where the ultrasound department is?" Roberta smiles and directs us upstairs.

"That's Schumann's *Fantasie*," Steve says and smiles as we snail it to the escalator and eventually land in the correct department. "I used to play that at Oberlin."

We shuffle up to the check-in counter. I frisk through his wallet for his insurance card and driver's license. After he's registered, we appropriate a couple of green vinyl seats positioned nearest the corridor that leads to the ultrasound department and settle in with outdated magazines. A waft of perfume from the woman sitting across from us inspires me to move us several rows away. I've no need right now for nausea and a headache. I flip through *The Week Magazine* and find a funny story about how dung beetles navigate by starlight. I hold it out to show Steve.

"Lucky buggers," I say. We'd had many a good laugh about my inability to follow any directions that included the words, "north, south, east or west."

"They can navigate by starlight!" I say. "I could have used their help that summer in the cornfield, remember?" He smiles and nods.

Not only can I not navigate by starlight, but my directional ineptitude almost got me fired when at sixteen I landed a summer job detasseling corn.

Removing tassels from the male stalks is necessary for the maintenance of superior hybrid corn, and it's most effectively done by hand. Detasseling is a hot and dirty job which paid well back then, more desirable than baby-sitting or waitressing. Anyway, that summer, five of my girlfriends and I were finally tall enough to qualify and got ourselves hired by the DeKalb Hybrid Corn company.

We arose at 4:00 a.m. and drove an hour to Geneseo, Illinois, to meet the crew. Our "driver" was a young man who led us each to a different section of the field to begin our work. The rows were tight; the leaves overlapped, scratching our bare arms. The corn soared over our heads, so even at 5'9" I had to stretch up on my tiptoes just to reach the tassels.

After the driver deposited me at the beginning of my row, he said, "Now all you have to do is stay in this row and pull off the tassels as fast as you can. I'll be back to check on you in an hour."

"No problem," I said, staring at his dimples. I was going to be the best damn detasseler he'd ever seen. I set off like a house afire.

I was fast, all right, flinging the tassels hither and yon, but when the driver came to check up on me, he hollered, "What are you *doing?*"

"What do you m-mean?" I stammered, out of breath, hot and dirty with cuts on my arms from the knife-sharp leaves.

"You're supposed to stay in a straight line—you're going diagonally across the field!" His face turned red, but not from the sun.

What? Afraid I'd be fired, I offered an anemic, "I'm sorry. I was going as fast as I could." He dragged me out of that row, found another and ordered me to start over. In my defense, the corn stalks were packed in so tight I couldn't tell one row from another.

If I'd been a dung beetle, this wouldn't have happened.

My job now is to keep up the banter with Steve, not betray my fear. I'm on high alert for any changes in him. I'm antsy for him to complete the ultrasound so I can call the social worker, the doctor, anyone, to help him.

"We'll get this over with, Honey, and when we're back in the room, I'm going to get you some help. It's not right that you're so confused." I pat his knee. He nods through a familiar foolish stare, the one that broadcasts to me he's in trouble.

A young nursing assistant finally appears and calls for Steve. We rise up, wounded soldiers stumbling into sick bay, and slowly make our way over to her. She leads us down the long tiled hall toward the ultrasound department, points to the waiting room for me and directs Steve to the changing cubicle where the gowns are kept.

"Uh," I say, "he can't do that by himself." I take him by the arm. We're as cramped in the paneled dressing room as we were in the United Airlines lavatory.

"You know, Steve, we have to stop meeting like this," I say. "How 'bout I strip you naked?"

"Don't make me laugh," he says and reaches for the grab bars. One button at a time, one pant leg at a time, one sock, one shoe. At last, he can slip into the gown with my help. I mistakenly fasten the ties in the back. We crack the door where the assistant is waiting to lead Steve off for his test. She glances at the ties and says, "Don't worry, I'll fix that."

I nod to the other woman in the waiting room, reach for the *New Yorker*. My eyes blur over *Shouts and Murmurs*, the words don't stick; my mind chirrs like an insect in distress. If I were a nail biter, I'd have had them all down to the quick by the time Steve is finished, an hour-and-a-half later.

We grab a taxi and arrive at our hotel in twenty minutes.

It's Noon. I escort an exhausted Steve to his room and help him undress so he can lie down after lunch. I snatch some leftovers from the fridge, ready a plate and a Glucerna—his favorite meal replacement drink—and bring it to him.

"Why don't you finish this while I eat and then call your social worker?" I rush to my room, shovel in some chicken salad, wash it down with green tea. If only he could get some Lactulose, I'm pretty sure his fog would lift. I don't know why Dr. Yilmaz didn't order an ammonia test.

I'm operating from my Nice Girl persona, not wanting to upset anyone who has the power to deny Steve a new liver. It's not a persona, really, just the way I was raised. Be kind, respectful, helpful, even. And, most importantly, never make a fuss. People don't like girls or women who make a fuss. Doctors especially don't like women who make a fuss. Perhaps Dr. Yilmaz thought that I, a mere woman, was out of line to even suggest he give Steve an ammonia test. I hope this is not a harbinger, flashing bright red.

★★★

During all the years I managed the therapy departments in centers for the rehabilitation of adults with physical disabilities—in-patient as well as out-patient—the social worker had always been the designated contact for the family. Since I've not been told otherwise, I assume Mary, the transplant social worker, will be Steve's care coordinator.

Later, I will recall a joke I once heard about the word, "assume"—it makes an "ass" out of "you and me."

Chapter Four

ONLY THE BEGINNING

Wednesday, January 14, 2015
At 12:30 p.m.

I call the number on Mary's card. After providing Steve's identifying information to the operator, I say, "Please tell Mary to call me back right away. Steve's confusion is getting worse and he can hardly function now. It's urgent that I talk with her." I leave my phone number.

At 1:30 p.m., having received no call, I make another urgent plea to the operator.

At 2:00 p.m., another social workers rings to tell me that Mary is busy but perhaps she, Maya, could help. I review my concerns again and tell her how urgent it is that Steve be tested and receive the medication.

She says, "I'll call Dr. Yilmaz's nurse, Andrea, and relay your message."

At 2:30 p.m., I leave my own message with Dr. Yilmaz's office—"Urgent, call me now!"

At 3:00 p.m. I'm frantic and I'm pissed. I worry that I won't reach anyone before they leave for the day. How can this be happening? We just saw these fucking people—why don't they call us back? I take deep slow breaths to thwart the hysteria crouching in my chest. I want so much to scream, but I was raised in the Midwest and steeped in the fine art of sucking it up.

I have no way of knowing how much or how often I will have to suck it up during the next four months. Or maybe I will eventually realize that I must stop the sucking up and lodge a complaint when it becomes obvious that no one is listening to me.

Jan phones again. My fear tumbles out. I tell her I'm doing the best I can, but I need to keep off the phone, just in case. "Love you, bye-bye."

Desperate, pacing, hyperventilating, it suddenly occurs to me to email Dan, our insurance company's nurse coordinator back in California who arranged the evaluation at this hospital for us.

I peek in on Steve—snoring. I snatch my purse and race to the business center, fire off an email.

> "Dear Dan,
>
> Thought I should tell you that Steve is getting quite confused—it's much worse since we came here. I have a call in to Dr. Yilmaz's assistant. I'm not sure if Steve's ammonia levels are going up or what, but I'm very concerned. I don't think he will be fit to travel on Friday. (Our original plan called for completing the evaluations by Friday and then flying home.)
>
> I might have to see if either his son or sister can fly in to be with him so I can go home and get things ready for us to be gone for up to six months. He's

not safe now to be left alone. Yesterday he stood in front of the bathroom mirror and couldn't figure out the buttons on his shirt. This morning, he mistook his shoe for a sock and had trouble understanding his appointment schedule, and other things. I hope they can do something about this.

I'll keep you posted.
Thanks, Rosie"

Seven minutes later, on my way out of the computer room, my cell phone rings. It's Dan.

"This is terrible!" he says. "You need to take Steve to the emergency room—right now!"

My breath catches. "Oh, crap. I'll go get him right away. Thank you!" I bolt to the elevators, heart pounding, fear unspooling. *What the fuck?* No one in the elevator meets my eyes.

I fly down the hallway, burst into my room, weeping, kicking myself.

Why didn't I think of that? If I can't even get this right, what's the rest of the journey going to be like? Up to now, I've been winging it; what if I'm really not up to this?

I shout, "Steve, Steve," as I slide through his adjoining door, wiping my eyes. "You've got to get up. I just talked to Dan and he said to take you to the ER. Now!" Steve slowly rolls over. The phone in my room rings. I rush to it.

"Hello," I say, panting.

"This is Andrea, Dr. Yilmaz's nurse. I understand there's a problem?"

"You might say," I holler. "I've been trying to reach you people for hours. Steve is more confused than ever. I'm pretty sure his ammonia has risen and he needs Lactulose which we don't have with us. He needs help, and none of you have called me back. I just got off the phone with Dan and he told me to take Steve to the emergency room."

"I'm very sorry this happened," she said. "My supervisor is going to have a talk with the person who took your messages. She didn't tell us they were urgent."

"Well, that doesn't help me now, does it?" I snapped. "Listen, I need you to call down to the ER and tell them one of your transplant patients is coming in and that they should see him right away!"

"Well, I'm not sure . . ." I slam down the phone and swivel toward Steve.

"Come on, Steve, we've got to boogie."

Down the hall, into the elevator, dash for the cab.

What if we're too late?

Chapter Five

THIS CAN'T BE HAPPENING

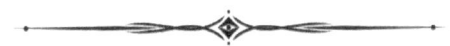

Wednesday, January 14, 2015
4:00 p.m.

M y heart pounds as the taxi swerves into the Emergency Entrance roundabout behind an ambulance. The temperature is dropping. Snow wisps around us, dusting the sidewalks, the cars, the bushes. Even so, I had asked the driver to hurry. Fighting to calm my breath, I pat Steve's thigh and say, "This is good, Steve, really good that Dan told us to come here. You just need some Lactulose, is all. You'll be fine in a jiffy." Deep inhale.

Don't scare him. Don't scare yourself.

A line of wheelchairs sits under the portico, oldster stock cars waiting for the starting gun. I flail myself out of the cab, dash up the slant, grab the sturdiest one, wheel it to the cab door. Slower than a slug in winter, I ease Steve's transfer into it. I strain to push all 230 pounds of him plus a tote bag up the ramp and into the waiting room, wheel him over to the check-in desk and set the brakes.

I fish around in his pack for his driver's license and insurance ID card. As soon as I open my mouth to the receptionist, I'm throttled with tears, the damn tears and shaky breath. I want to scream, *Would someone goddammit please help me??!! My husband is dying, for chrissakes!*

Swiping my nose on the back of my hand, chewing my lip and sorting my breath, I try to explain to the clerk what is going on. "Did you get a call from Andrea?" He shakes his head. He notes Steve's information in his computer and asks us to take a seat. The chilly waiting room is already crowded with slumping, coughing patients, their miseries palpable. On the walls, not even the prominent paintings of Georgia O'Keefe flowers can cheer me up.

"This is urgent," I say, shifting my weight from one foot to another. "How long will it be before he's seen?"

"They'll get to him as soon as they can, ma'am." He hands over Steve's identification and insurance cards to me. I slip them back into Steve's pack.

I wheel Steve into a quiet corner, far away from the blathering TV's and the other sick desperate people. We can't afford to contract anything now. I settle into one of the padded vinyl seats next to Steve and reach for his hand. The light snow melt from our shoes glistens in tiny puddles at our feet.

"OK, Sweetheart," I say and sigh. "I'm sure they'll see you soon. They'd better if they want to keep their contract with our insurance carrier! Dan was pretty pissed." I blink around at the sick and wounded, as I kiss him on the check. "You're going to be fine, Honey. You just need some Lactulose."

My anger at Dr. Yilmaz metastasizes into rage. If he had listened to me and ordered a blood test to check his ammonia level, I'm certain we wouldn't need to be here.

If this is the best they can do during the evaluation week, how can I possibly trust them with Steve's transplant?

I reach into my bag, pull out my pink fleece jacket and shrug into it. Steve runs hot and is comfortable in his short-sleeved Hawaiian shirt. Fifteen minutes pass. Nothing. My insides are coiled, fixing to strike at the nearest nurse. My impulse is to grab her by the stethoscope and scream, "You've got *do* something! Now!"

One by one, patients are called by a nurse ("Mr. Jessup, Mr. Jessup,") standing near the entrance to the treatment area.

Fuck Mr. Jessup and the horse he rode in on.

Twenty minutes later, still staring at the same page in *Newsweek,* nothing. I tell Steve I'm going to check with the triage nurse.

He shakes himself awake. "Please don't piss them off," he says, gripping the arms of his wheelchair.

This raises my ire. "Don't worry, Steve, I'll be fine. But you need help right now, and I'll do whatever it takes to get it," I say. His brow furrows. I pat his hand and kiss him. "I'll try to be nice."

That old shibboleth again— "Be nice." Seldom applied to boys, but all the time to girls. Which means just you shut up and do what you're told and don't upset any adult, ever. You're expected to sacrifice your wishes and needs on the altar of keeping everyone else happy.

In this rigged game, your turn seldom comes.

I stand up, affix my best anodyne smile, and wait patiently in the triage area where the nurse is entering information into her computer. I notice "Nancy" stamped on her name tag.

Finally, she looks up. "Yes?" she says, still typing.

"I know you're very busy, Nancy, but I just wanted to find out when Steve will be seen. Steve West. He's a liver transplant patient and he's really sick right now. I think his ammonia level is up." My voice rises. I feel like a fool for tearing up.

The nurse stops typing and glances over at Steve.

"Soon, ma'am. We'll get to him as soon as we can." Typing resumes.

Soon is not good enough. Soon is too late. Soon is bullshit.

"Thank you," I say and scuff back to Steve. He's dozing in his chair. Oh, would that I, too, could nap right now.

Forty-five minutes later, at 6:30 p.m., Steve's name is called, "West? Mr. Steven West?" The nurse awaits near the treatment room door. I thrust up my waving hand—*over here! Here he is!*

"Wake up, Honey," I whisper and nudge him as I scoot around to the back of his wheelchair and unlock the brakes. I wheel him as fast as I can toward the nurse.

Oh, please God, let there be help.

"Thank you," I say to her. "He's quite sick." The familiar fragrance of disinfectant quirks my nose. I'm caught by the distinctive sounds of an Emergency Room: a patient moaning; bells dinging; the PA system crying out, "Dr. Rach, please come to the ER, Dr. Rach, come to the ER." Assistants high stepping it from one patient to another. Metal screeching up on metal as curtains are being slithered to and fro along steel rods.

The nurse directs us to the first room on the right and assists Steve with his transfer from the wheelchair to the bed. Two other younger nurses buzz in, all smiles.

"Hi, Mr. West. My name is Sheila and this is Maggie," two blond forty-somethings with weary, but interested eyes. "What can we do for you today?" They look upon him with kindness.

"Well, uh," he says and stares at me. A lost puppy yearning for a hug and a bone.

"He's a liver transplant patient," I say, "and he's very confused. He's been on Xifaxan but I don't think it's doing the job of keeping his ammonia level down. I'm pretty sure he needs some Lactulose. We're from California, didn't bring any with us." I blow my nose to keep from crying. "We'd been told by his liver doc at home that we shouldn't mix those two meds."

"Got it," Maggie says. "Let's get you ready, Mr. West, and then draw some blood to find out what's going on. Is that OK?"

They set to work, gowning him in no time, hooking him up to a monitor, drawing blood, whisking the tubes off to the lab.

I've already collapsed into a chair, relieved for them to take over. Steve is an unreliable narrator; so I have to fill in all the information he cannot summon through his fog.

I push up and stand by his side, caress his hand. "You're going to be fine now, Honey. They'll get you some Lactulose, so you'll feel much better in no time!"

"I hope so." His wan smile breaks my heart.

I lean down to kiss him. "I know so." I've been up since 5:30 a.m. and droop back to the chair, depleted, a marionette with no strings. Steve dozes.

Forty minutes later, a tall, blond man wearing round metal-framed eyeglasses, enters the room, smiling. He extends his hand and says, "I'm Dr. Schafer. I'm the surgical resident on call, and I'll be taking care of your husband."

"Thanks," I say. "Nice to meet you." I release his hand. "Have the ammonia results come back yet?"

"As a matter of fact, they have. The level is very high at 97, so we are going to start him on some Lactulose." (Normal range for ammonia is 10-50).

"Oh, thank God," I say. "I thought the Xifaxan was supposed to take care of all of this."

"Not always," he says and moves toward Steve who is sleeping. He leans near the bed. "Hi, Mr. West, can you wake up for me?"

Steve opens his eyes. I spring up and move over to him. "This is Dr. Schafer, Honey, he's going to help you. He's ordered some Lactulose."

"Oh," he says and smiles. "Hi." Steve's good nature seldom fails him, even now.

Dr. Schafer says, "Can I have a look at your belly?"

"Sure," Steve says and fumbles with his gown.

"That's OK, I've got it," he says and lifts it up over Steve's abdomen.

"I see you've got some ascites here—have they tapped this for you?"

Steve looks over at me, questioning. Tapping means sticking a needle into his abdomen to drain the fluid, not unlike tapping a beer keg.

"No," I say, "our GI doctor at home didn't want to do that before we left, said he'd leave that up to the transplant doctors here." I blew my nose and shoved the tissue into my jacket pocket.

Another nurse, Stacey, arrives with the Lactulose in a small measured cup, gives him his first dose. *Thank you, Jesus!*

Dr. Schafer says, "I'm going to go look at your records some more, Mr. West. I will be right back."

We're all alone now. "You're going to be right as rain in no time, Steve. I'm so relieved we came here." Steve nods and closes his eyes.

Dr. Schafer returns and says, "I think we should do a CAT scan."

"Why is that?"

"Just to make sure there isn't anything else going on."

"I'm sure he'll feel better now that he's had his Lactulose," I say, my voice rising in uncertainty.

"We'll wait and see." He leaves the room.

Within 45 minutes, Steve is talking like his old self. It is now 8:30 p.m.

"You're back, Honey. How do you feel?"

Please, please be normal again.

"Much better." I ease my hip onto his bed, give him a twisted ersatz hug.

Dr. Schafer returns and says, "We decided not to do a CAT scan, after all, but I think it best if we keep him overnight."

"Why is that?" I say and toss up my hands.

"Just to be careful. And also, so we can finish all his evaluations while he's in the hospital. I'll order a bed," he says and leaves. I'm not sure this is necessary, but I'm not the doctor, so—

At 9:30 p.m., I ask Stacey, "What about the bed?" Steve has been asleep for an hour or so.

"They have to get it ready on the transplant unit. I'll let you know when he can be moved," she says and dashes back out the door. I admire anyone who becomes a nurse. They so often do not get the credit they deserve.

It is 10:20 p.m. I am so damn tired that I consider leaving Steve in the care of the doctors and nurses and returning to the hotel to sleep. 5:30 a.m. feels like eons ago.

Stacey breezes back in and says, "Should be any time now, but before he goes to the transplant floor, I have to give him a shot of heparin." She turns around and leaves.

I'm groggy, but within a few seconds, one sleepy neuron fires, then another, then another and pretty soon a swarm is buzzing, lighting up my brain . . . *What the hell?*

"I'll be right back, Steve!" I whirl around and shove out the door.

I sprint down the hall, hollering, "Stacey, Stacey!" I skid to a stop. "Does the doctor know Steve has only 30,000 platelets?" I'm panting now. "I don't think it's safe for him to get a blood thinner right now!"

In a normal human, platelet levels vary from 150,000 to 450,000. Platelets are those little critters that help the blood to clot. Heparin is a powerful blood thinner and with Steve's already low platelets, I'm afraid a bolus of heparin might endanger him. I can't let them take that chance.

Her face registers no concern. "I'll ask him."

Isn't that something a nurse should have known about?

I whip around and book it back to Steve's door just in time to head off another nurse carrying a large syringe, but before he can enter Steve's room, I say, out of breath, "Uh, is that heparin?"

"Yes," he says, annoyed. *Who is this crazy woman getting in my way?*

"No! No!" I say too loudly. "You're not giving that to him." I move to block him from the doorway. *I'll drop you right here if you move any closer.*

"I just talked with Stacey. She needs to make sure Dr. Schafer is aware that Steve has only 30,000 platelets."

Jesus, what kind of place is this? What if I'd gone back to the hotel? He might be dead by morning.

Chapter Six

WAS THIS A BAD IDEA?

Wednesday, January 14, 2015
11:00 p.m.

S queaky wheels scream me awake. The chair in the ER was
not comfortable, but exhaustion triumphed over pain. The
transport attendant arrived with a new bed to wheel Steve to the
second floor transplant unit. I trail along with our belongings
clutched to my chest, spilling over my arms.

Exhausted and shaking. I had seriously considered leaving last
night, believing Steve was in safe hands and that I could go to
the hotel to get some rest. Safe hands? Ha! The thought that he
might have died from the heparin shot before he could even have
a chance at a transplant lands in my stomach with a thud. I could
never have lived with myself.

Rolling from the service elevator toward Steve's room, we
pass several others, some with doors open. I'm a scout doing
recon, gawking into every room. Steve will stay on this unit
after his transplant, assuming he passes all their tests and they
don't try to kill him again. How bad do the patients look? Are

family members distressed or relaxed? Do the nurses seem nice or cranky? Is the unit smelly?

The attendant hastens Steve's bed through the hallway. Bells are dinging. The PA system is calling for "Dr. Santiago, Dr. Santiago, please call extension 513." The night crew is mopping the floors but make way for us. He wheels Steve into a room where his new nurse awaits. Sterile off-white walls with a few scattered photos of flowers and a television attached to a swinging arm screwed high to the ceiling.

"Hello, Mr. West," the nurse says to Steve and takes over the bed from the attendant. He carefully maneuvers it into its proper place and locks down the wheels.

"I'm David," he says with a smile, "and I'll be your nurse until early morning." Steve nods. I wave. "We're going to get you all set up for the night." He quickly slips Steve into a fresh gown and hooks him up to oxygen, heart monitor, IV, and then begins to draw blood.

I dump our belongings onto the green plaid vinyl window seat and plop down, my right foot jiggling.

When David finishes his set-up, I stand and extend my hand, "Hi. I'm Steve's wife. I would like to talk to you about heparin, if I may." He gives it a brief, warm shake.

Another nurse, wearing Mickey Mouse tennies, pops in and says, "Have you seen Dr. Peterson on the unit tonight?"

"No," Dave says, "I don't think so." Mickey Mouse tennies closes the door.

"Sorry about that," he says. "I know the order for heparin has been cancelled." David stands about 5'10", slim but muscled, curly dark hair, wide smile. Barely 30, I'd guess.

"Can you please tell me who prescribed that?" I ask, pursing my lips to keep my agita at bay.

"Sure, let's see," he says and turns to the computer, waving me close.

I step to his side as he mouses through all the entries, points to the screen and says, "It was Dr. Schafer."

"I don't know why he did that when Steve had only 30,000 platelets," I sigh and rub my forehead. "That could have been dangerous. Would you please make sure that there's no longer an order for heparin anywhere in Steve's file? We had a close call earlier tonight, as I'm sure you know, and we can't afford another screw-up." I cross my arms over my chest, mostly to keep warm.

David continues scrolling through the entire online record and assures me the order has been deleted. He turns around and says, reassuringly, "That won't happen again. Just so you know, they often prescribe heparin for liver transplant patients because they have to be lying in bed for so long."

"Well then, they all must have more platelets than Steve does."

Suddenly, a piercing unintelligible sound of indeterminate origin invades the room.

"What the heck is that?" I say, cringing.

"That's one of our patients next door," he says and shrugs his shoulders. "He's having trouble with his meds. They have to give them high doses of steroids right after surgery and some people don't tolerate that."

"Will he get better?" Worry gathers in my voice. I glance toward Steve who is buried under the covers and snoring.

"Yes. He just has to stay on it for a few more days to protect his transplant," he says as he tidies up his work station. The howling subsides.

"Ah. Well, maybe we could keep the door closed so he doesn't wake Steve if he screams again?"

Is there nothing I can control?

As soon as David finishes his prep work, I lean in and kiss Steve. "Looks like you're going to be in good hands tonight, Honey. I'm heading back to the hotel to get some sleep."

"OK." He rolls over and resumes snoring. Dodging a near-death bullet can exhaust a fella. I don my jacket, fasten my fanny pack, hook my arm through the handles of my tote bag and slow walk to the door.

"Good-night, David," I say with a smile wider than usual, "and thanks."

He seems nice. He seems competent. But then, so did Dr. Schafer. Oh, crap, should I stay with him? But where could I sleep? The window seat won't allow me to stretch out. My neck and back can't tolerate that. I'm already in a lot of pain from dozing in that chair. My beloved chiropractor is almost 2,000 miles away. There's nothing to do but return to my comfy bed in the hotel and pray Steve will be OK.

"Sure thing. I'll take good care of him," he says as I leave and pull the door behind me.

Fatigue overrides my concern. Without sleep, I am nothing.

Thursday, January 15, 2015
8:30 a.m.

I phone Steve, eager to hear his voice. After yesterday's snafu I'm loath to ever leave him, but last night I had little choice if I wanted to be prepared for who-knows-what hurdles we might face today. Friday can't come soon enough to whisk him away to the safety of home.

"Hi," Steve says, clearing the sleep from his throat.

"Hello, Sweetheart. Apparently, they managed not to kill you last night." *Ha.*

"No. I'm fine. David was great. I have a new nurse this morning, Karen."

"God, am I relieved. Look, I need to sleep in a little longer. I'll be in around noon. I have a bunch of things I need to do before I come over—emails to family, get some take-out. Is that OK?"

"Sure. I'm fine." It's that sweet baritone voice that won me over when I first met him. It never ceases to thrill when I hear him on the phone.

"All right, Sweets. See you later. You've got my cell number, so call me if anything comes up."

You hang up the phone and now, finally alone, you can cry—big fat sobbing, slobbering tears. You don't know how much more of this you can take, and they're not even done with his evals. You're horrified about yesterday and last night. If you hadn't known what heparin was, and if you'd not stayed with him, well . . . you might not be having a Steve to bring home with you on Friday.

I cry and doze and cry and doze. *How in the hell am I going to make it through his transplant?* Assuming he lives long enough to get one.

I finally leave the bed, don my black slacks, white fuzzy sweater and dark blue jacket, wanting to look friendly, but not like a pushover. I grab two hard-boiled eggs from the fridge, slug down some ibuprofen and plod off to the Business Center to email Steve's family and friends. What do I say? *Well, so far so good. They've tried to kill him only once . . . can't wait to see how the rest of the week unfolds, will keep in touch, bye bye, love.*

I call Dan. He picks up right away.

"How are you?" he says, concern in his voice.

"Not great, Dan." The entire debacle spills out—how we ended up in the ER because no one returned my calls about Steve's confusion, and then the heparin caper.

"This is terrible." I hear a catch in his breath.

"Yes, it is, it is," I say and scoot my chair closer to the desk. "So tell me something, Dan, assuming he lives through the week, why should I bring him back here for a transplant?"

"Right. Well, for one, they have access to more organs in that region than we have in California. And, just as important, the surgeons there are excellent. Our patients have gotten very good results."

"Well, that's nice, but many of the other staff don't seem to know what the hell they're doing." I tug at my bangs. "There's no excuse for this level of incompetence."

"We've had some issues with them, yes, and I've reported your problems to my superiors who have reported to their managers. They have promised me they are working on better case management procedures."

"In what century might we expect that?" I say, making no effort to hide the sarcasm.

"You could, if you want, go check out two other hospitals we have contracts with."

"You mean drag Steve all over the country?" I start scratching my head. "Start with new people and . . . ?"`

I tear up, slump in my chair, my spine an S-curve of defeat.

"Dan. I'm exhausted," I say, sighing with some force. "Steve is exhausted and he's very sick. I don't think either of us could survive. He needs a new liver NOW!"

"I agree. I've already talked to the individuals on the liver transplant team and told them about what you've gone through, and that I am not happy about that. One of them will probably contact you before you leave."

"Can't wait, but I have to tell you, Dan, I'm not going to promise to be nice."

You're beginning to feel a seismic shift—wriggling away from the straightjacket you grew up in where you didn't dare talk back to anyone, would never question the wisdom of your physician, and would rather die than be thought rude. Well.

You can see now that being nice can get you killed, or worse yet, someone you love could die.

Time for your inner tomboy to swing for the fences.

Thank goodness for Dan. A former transplant nurse, he now coordinates all the out-of-state referrals for our health plan. Our very own concierge.

Bad enough that they're making this week hell, but, assuming Steve gets listed, I must fly Steve home and arrange for us to be away for up to six months while we live somewhere near the hospital, waiting for his new liver. This means packing all the stuff we will need while we're gone, sending much of it ahead; arranging for a good cat caretaker for our two cats, one of whom needs asthma medication every other day; figuring out how to get our bills paid, our mail sorted and goodness knows what else. My breath is spiraling out of control; hyperventilation ready to pounce. Must stop, take a breath before I pass out. I need to tuck away those worries so I can buck up and speed Steve the hell home tomorrow.

I hit *send* on an email to his family and friends. "Yes, well, we've had a few glitches, but he's doing fine, and we hope to finish up the evals in time to return on Friday." No sense telling them the truth; nothing they could do.

I taxi to the hospital, indulge in my daily pilgrimage to the cafeteria where I line up behind nurses and doctors in search of a heart-healthy meal. Snag two non-offending sandwiches (I can always scrape off the mayo) and two glasses of iced tea. I need to eat pretty much all the time to keep my energy up.

I tread up the tiled staircase, preferring to walk in lieu of taking the elevator. Must keep up some semblance of fitness. I gaze at the portraits of all the hospital's previous presidents lining the dusty peach wall, all men, all grim-looking. I mull over Dan's comments about the hospital's excellent surgeons and our option to visit other hospitals. Out of the question. We have to hope against hope, assuming he's accepted for a transplant, that the surgery will go as Dan has described.

What will we do if he's not accepted?

Steve's sister Jan said she'd fly out from Maine to be with us after the transplant, assuming he gets one. His son Landon plans to join us after that. My zombie brain is now on overload, thinking about all that could go wrong. I can't wait for us to make a break for it tomorrow.

I slow walk my way past the other patient rooms again. How are they doing this morning? I see a few smiles, but most faces are drained and drawn. In one small family waiting room, I notice several sleeping bags on the floor, cocoons with no movement discernible. On the low coffee table lay empty Coke cans, Snickers wrappers. McDonald's abandoned fries packets lie strewn about like so much wreckage on the side of the road. This is the stuff normal people eat when they're stressed.

"Hey, Honey," I say as I push open the door to Steve's room, and wave to the nurse.

"You must be Karen." I walk up to her, shake her hand. "I hope he's behaving."

"No. He's pretty much been a bear," she says, exuding kindness and good will.

"Good. Now I know he's feeling better," I say and walk over to give him a kiss.

I stash my bags in the closet and pull out a book, wave it in the air.

"I brought your book, Honey, not that you'll have time to read it," and set it on his bed. *The English Language*, by David Crystal, one of Steve's faves. He picks it up and smiles.

"So. What's the platelet count today?" I ask Karen.

"About the same, holding steady. He's had a CAT scan and ultrasound already this morning. And, of course, more blood work."

"There's probably not an inch of you they haven't examined, Steve."

"True enough," says Karen. "They want to make absolutely sure he's able to tolerate the procedure, which is pretty tough."

"So am I," says Steve. He's right about that. He spent his time on the farm milking cows, plowing fields, slinging hay bales "to hell and gone," as he is fond of saying, and working on a construction gang in the summers. When he moved in with me many years ago, he carried his sofa on his back up a flight of seventeen stairs. Who does that?

Thursday passes quickly. I nap on the window seat, designed for just such a purpose. I'm turned on my side, cuddled up with a pillow and a blanket Karen has given me. I keep one ear cocked to the goings on. I can lie in this position for only 30 minutes at a time before my back and neck kick up a fuss. Karen's obvious caring and competence help me relax.

Around 4:00, I receive a call from a woman named Sally who says she will be Steve's transplant coordinator. She says she's talked with Dan and with her own supervisor about the phone problem, insists it was unfortunate that I never told the operator the call was "urgent."

My brain wakes up. Again? "Excuse me?" I say. "I made at least three calls in the afternoon and each time I told the operator I needed to speak to someone now, that it was urgent."

"That's not what she said," says Sally.

I quickly do a mental review of my phone calls to the operator. I know damn well I said it was urgent that someone should get back to me. What's going on? Is gaslighting now their new case management protocol? I head toward the door and out into the hall. I move away from the patient rooms and into an alcove by a window.

"Why the hell do you think I kept calling? Here we are, having flown all the way from California, don't know anyone, don't know how your system works, were never told what to do in case of an emergency while we're here, and I had to call Dan in California for advice? How do you explain that?"

"Well, like I said, the operator insists you never used the word 'urgent.'"

"You know, we wouldn't be in this situation if either Mary, the social worker, or Dr. Yilmaz had listened to me on that first day. I told them how confused Steve was, more so than at home and that he probably needed some Lactulose. If they had only listened to me, we wouldn't be having this discussion, and Steve wouldn't have damn near been killed in your fucking ER!"

"I'm very sorry about all this," she says.

I'm not feeling it. "Sorry? You're sorry?"

"I'd like to make an appointment to visit with you and Steve tomorrow," she says.

"I don't know why, but you'll have to come in the morning because we're flying home at 4:00."

"OK. How about 9:00 a.m.?"

"Fine," I say and hang up.

Blaming me? Really?

★★★

My blood is boiling. I seldom get this angry about anything, but if they think I will roll over and say I'm sorry when I did nothing wrong, then they've got another think coming.

Buried deep in my repertoire is the memory of how I stood up, finally, to my rageaholic father who thought it was perfectly within his right, without warning, to fire off his backhand across the side of my head, with no care for the damage it might inflict.

After many years of his abuse, I finally snapped—one of those, "I'm mad as hell and I'm not going to take it anymore" moments from a male actor in an old movie. He, of course, was a man and therefore sanctified by his audience for his outbursts.

A woman would have been hauled off to the loony bin.

By the time I turned sixteen, I was already 5'9," the high school volleyball champ, full of spring and fire. One evening, Dad, itching for another fight, stomped into the dining room and ordered me to leave my Latin assignment unfinished and go to bed. "And I mean now, Dunce!" Neither my mom nor my brother were home.

"No," I snapped, "I'm not coming. I've got things to do." My eyes were on my text, but my attention was on my dad. My mouth was dry, my hands shaking. This was going to end right here, right now.

Out of the corner of my eye, I saw his tremble begin, and as I shot up, I shoved back the dining room chair so hard it slammed into Mom's china cabinet, rattling the few pieces of good china she owned.

We squared off on the other side of the table. I knew he was fixin' to take a swing, but instead of running out of the house as usual, I planted my feet on Mom's new rose-colored carpet, stretched out my spine like they tell you to do if you're confronted by a cougar, readied my tomboy fists and screamed, "Don't you EVER hit me again!"

I scared myself half out of my wits.

He stopped, his eyes wild with disbelief. He was tall and menacing, but I had less to lose, and I knew I could take him.

Good thing I didn't know how to use my brother's twelve-gauge shotgun or my father could have joined that other father from several towns away in having his head blown off by his angry teenager. I stared as his rage turned to worry, then defeat. His skinny arms loosened and dropped by his sides as he rushed out the back door, saying, "Ah, shit."

He. Never. Hit. Me. Again.

One day I may need to call upon the cussedness of that 16 year-old girl for help.

Friday, January 16, 2015
9:00 a.m.

Sally, the transplant nurse coordinator, knocks on the door, enters the room and introduces herself to Steve and me. She's short, about fifty with thinning gray hair. I had decided overnight that I would bite my tongue and play along; didn't want them rejecting Steve because of me. She brings with her a large three-ring binder bulging with documents. I hold my tongue.

We should have been given this notebook on our first day.

We proceed to have a civil discussion as she flips through the book, section by section. Says she's sorry we didn't get the information first thing on Monday from the social worker.

Around 10:00 a.m., a nurse practitioner, James, hustles into the room, walks over to Steve.

"Mr. West?" he asks. Steve nods. I rise up and stand by the bed. "I need to tell you, Mr. West, that some of your tests came back suspicious for blood cancer. We're repeating them to make sure, but the results won't be available until much later today."

Sally sets the notebook on the window seat, waves and scoots out the door.

"Oh no," I say, "We're supposed to fly home today at 4:00 p.m." *Crap.*

James goes on, "We can't finish Mr. West's evaluation and make a decision about his listing status until we know for sure that the tests are negative. It sometimes happens that we get false positives. But until we know for sure —"

Not now! Not when we're so close.

I take a few deep breaths, look over at Steve and say, "I gotta go call Dan and let him know we can't fly out today. I'll see if he can help us get a flight for tomorrow." I race out of the room.

"Don't worry," Dan says. "I'm on it. I'll call you back when I have something to recommend."

Please God, even though I don't believe in you very much, can you deliver us from this fresh hell?

At 4:00 p.m. the nurse practitioner returns to notify us that the transplant committee has met and they have decided to "list" Steve. The most beautiful word in the English language: "list." It means he has been officially accepted for a transplant and put on their waiting list. What a relief. He's going to get a new liver!

"Go home," James says "and arrange everything so you can return soon. We will be in touch."

"I assume then that he doesn't have lymphoma?" I can barely eke out the question.

He shakes his head. "Sorry about that. The first tests were false positive. It happens."

I have no words.

Chapter Seven

OUTTA HERE!

Saturday, January 17, 2015
4:00 a.m.

Steve and I have been running bases on wobbly legs for the past five days, finally skidding into home plate on Friday with the umpire yelling, "Safe!"

I've completed the packing and am organizing everything for our trip back to California, including Steve, who simply cannot hurry. I tell him, "Time to blow this pop stand, baby!"

We slide into the cab at 5:30. Chilly with snow still mucking up the ground. Deafening shriek of planes flying overhead as we draw near the airport at 6:30. Shivering and stomping our feet, the taxi idles at the curb, spewing exhaust fumes while the driver unloads our bags and thanks me for the tip. We check two of our bags at the United Airlines curb counter and ask for help securing motorized transport to the gate. We climb on as quickly as we can, given Steve's lack of energy, and float away on the quiet hush of the electric cart. The airport is warmer than it needs to be. We shrug out of our jackets as we zoom around the other weary travelers, pass by restaurants with hungry breakfast lines, glitzy gift shops and staid newsstands. No time to stop at Starbucks. When we arrive at the gate, the agent very kindly escorts us to the front of the boarding line after I detail Steve's medical condition, point to his medic alert necklace and hand over our passes.

"Of course," she says. "No problem."

We don our jackets again and wrestle our bags as we slowly tortoise our way down the aisle, welcomed by the steady thrum of the air conditioner. Our seats are near the lavatory. A cute flight attendant named Brad approaches and says, "Thank you for flying United. Here, let me help you with your carry ons." I move us out of the way as he crams many of our belongings into the overhead bin, the rest under the seats in front of us.

"Thanks so much for your help," I say. He nods and smiles, turns and walks away. Nice buns.

We're finally, happily tucked into our seats. I close my eyes, slump back and sigh. *Please let us get home safely*, I pray to no entity in particular. I need to relax, read my CIA thriller for the next few hours, inhabit a world where there's order, where good guys prevail and the bad guys are laid to waste.

I rest my hand on Steve's arm. "We made it, Honey, we made it." He nods with an exhausted smile.

I bend down and rifle through my carry-on, pull out my plastic bottle of iced tea, a baggie loaded with cashews and Karen Cleveland's latest spy novel. Steady them on my lap until we can open up our tray tables.

The remaining travelers trudge up the aisle, scanning for vacancies. We pray that no one covets our window seat. I cast surreptitious glances at them, imagine stories of their lives as they chatter on their cell phones, struggle and swear at their carry ons and slurp their drinks as they pass.

Young twenty-something redhead, clutching a pillow to her chest, tears in her eyes. Might have just lost her mother. Oh, wait. Her ring finger is bereft of ring. In its place a white band of flesh encircled by tan. Might have abandoned her boyfriend at the altar, or vice versa.

Florid-faced heavyset man, lumbering, wipes sweat from his forehead, might have forgotten his blood pressure meds, possibly headed for a heart attack, hopefully not on this flight.

Old woman, stepping lively with her joking grandson, waving his inflated dinosaur at everyone he passes, happy to be alive.

No one appears as if they need a transplant.

"Everything's going to be fine, now," I say to Steve, with more hope than I actually harbor. "We can play with our kitties again, get some rest, then ready up for the return trip. The next time we fly home, you'll be wearing a new liver. Can you believe that? A miracle."

As presented to us upon Steve's discharge from the transplant unit, the plan is for Steve to return to the hospital once his MELD score rises to 22, no idea how soon that will be. Steve's score has been hovering between 19 and 21 for several months.

The MELD (model for end-stage liver disease) score provides an estimate of a patient's chances for surviving without a transplant over the next three months. The MELD ranges from six to forty, based on a formula incorporating three particular lab values—bilirubin, INR and creatinine. Bilirubin is a yellowish pigment made from the breakdown of red blood cells. INR is a test of the body's blood clotting ability. Creatinine is a measure of kidney function. The three values are entered into a specialized formula which yield the MELD score.

The higher the number, the higher the priority for a patient to receive a transplant. Also, the higher the number, the greater the likelihood the patient will die without it.

Steve begins to doze. He's not well. His abdomen is growing. I'm relieved their docs decided not to tap his belly to drain his ascites. They wanted to leave it up to our trusted physician back home. It's going to be hell again to wrestle him in and out of the bathroom during the next several hours and to guide him during the plane change. His auditory processing is not what it needs to be, even with his Lactulose and Xifaxin. I must speak very slowly and distinctly and wait for evidence of his understanding. The ticket agents assured us an attendant would be waiting for us with a wheelchair in Phoenix, and that the new gate would be close by. They're kind and are doing their best to make this trip work for us.

Can't wait to touch down in San Francisco.

The usual nuisances accompanying air travel seem trivial in comparison to the past four days. Steve is alive. I am alive. The rest is already receding into story, as if we had just emerged from someone else's nightmare.

Safe at home.

As soon as we open the front door, Billy, our strawberry blond mush cat, climbs out of his favorite plush bed near the fireplace and rushes up to Steve who hoists him up to his chest.

"Hey there, good buddy," Steve says. I'm sure our neighbors can hear Billy's freight train rumble of a purr. These boys have been bonded ever since we met Billy at the homeless cat colony I've taken care of for 15 years. Sugar, my Siamese mix, doesn't exist, at least not right now. Mommy must be punished. She'll stroll in from her hiding place in an hour or so. Does it every time I go away. Kitties do not like to have their beloved routines upset.

Humans are not much different. Traveling can be fun, even when things don't go as planned, but traveling with the life-threatening illness of one's beloved, well, let's just say that's not funny. I scan the room and notice that our neighbor, Mary Lou, has done a yeoman's job of keeping the litter boxes clean. Nothing worse than coming home to the smell of cat piss.

Our long-time friends, Scott and his wife Angie, fetched us at the airport, ferried us home and kindly brought in all our luggage and associated possessions. I met them years ago when I dated Scott's father. After we broke up, they made it clear that they still wanted me to be part of their family. They very graciously adopted Steve soon after he and I met. After hugging and thanking them, we say good-bye with a promise to treat them to dinner soon.

I unpack the absolute minimum—toothbrush, paste, floss and face soap for me; nighttime drugs for Steve—and abandon the suitcases in the living room for attention later. In his bedroom, Steve and I labor more than twenty minutes to remove his suspenders, trousers, shirt and pressure socks. Soon after I tuck him into bed, Billy sneaks in and hops up.

"Hello, there, Mr. Billster," says Steve and begins petting him under his chin. "Miss me?" They soon drift off and start snoring together—an antiphonal sing.

Sunday, January 18, 2015
9:00 a.m.

Hung over from worry and travel, I slide into my favorite sweats and slowly trudge to the kitchen for some eggs and toast, do a desultory flip through the mail Mary Lou has collected and stacked on the counter, and scuff out to the living room. The suitcases will have to wait until Steve arises. Even though he is ill, Steve is still stronger than me. All those years of baling hay, plowing fields on the family farm and working construction during the summers have paid off. Bumping into one of Steve's thighs is like crashing into a telephone pole.

I'm grateful we have returned to the land of redwood trees—nine stately friends guard the sidewalks near our home. Two sizeable windows in the living room shower us with an intimate view of their green branches waving in the breeze, welcoming us home. It's cold outside by California standards, 59°, but no snow. I set the thermostat to a comfortable 70° and listen for it to click on.

Sugar finally appears, my time of punishment apparently having ended. I swing her up to my chest and nuzzle her soft fur. "Well hello, Darling. I thought you were never going to speak to me again." She stares at me with her azure eyes, wants to make sure it's really me and not some stranger bent on kidnapping.

We proceed upstairs to my writing loft where, to her delight, her favorite lap soon appears, inviting her to hop aboard so she can wind herself into a ball while I email friends and family: "Hooray, we're home, we're fine, we're tired, more later. Thanks for everything." I check my answering machine, delete the mostly robo calls.

Down to the kitchen, trailed by my kitty, I set out some Fancy Feast. Off to the living room. Check the coffee table and sift through a few packages Mary Lou has kept for us. Nothing important except for a new set of bra straps.

I flop onto the sofa, lie back, my mind buzzing with all the things we, or rather I, need to get done before we can return for Steve's transplant. His surgeon told us we might be away for as long as six months while we wait for a new liver.

I am haunted by the fear that Steve might not last for six more months.

First thing, I've got to see Dr. Chris Nizer. His treatment is the one true relief I can count on for most of my pain, at least for a while, until I bend or twist or lift something I shouldn't.

In the meantime, I've got to kick start myself into activity when I'd rather treat my body to a month of bed rest. I sigh and cuddle up with the teal afghan our neighbor Shirley made for us before we left.

I know that Dan has communicated our problems to the transplant staff and hope that will have made a difference by the time we return to their care. For the time being, I'm just going to pretend that that is so. Of course we'll be fine. The hospital has a reputation for excellence, does it not?

Dissociation has a lot to recommend it—a two-dollar word for the cognitive-emotional state in which a person divides and stuffs all manner of unwanted feelings, memories and knowledge into mental box cars. While the cars may be traveling down the same track, each one has scant awareness of or communication with the others.

I must trust Dan's judgment about the transplant surgeons—that they're outstanding and that Steve will live long thereafter because of an excellent result. We have already met one of them—blond-mopped Dr. Anthony. He was very matter-of-fact about explaining the procedure, said he transplants two or more patients a day. His confidence calmed me. He told us that one of their surgeons actually flies to another hospital in the region when they become informed of a donation. The surgeons do the harvesting themselves, so they know ahead of time the quality of the organ they're bringing back, as well as the medical history and condition of the donor. I knew it was important for him to describe these things to us, but in the middle of his presentation, nausea set in. The idea of someone cutting open my sweetheart and installing a cadaver's liver roiled my own guts in sympathy. I had to subtly put on the brakes by telling him that that was all the info we needed right then, thank you very much. He handed over his card and invited us to call any time.

Monday, January 19, 2015
11:00 a.m.

Sitting at my desk in my writing loft, catching up on emails. Phone call from Janice Olsen, Quality Assurance Coordinator for our health plan.

We often screen our calls before answering, but when I hear her announcing her name and position, I rush to the phone, trying to keep calm, but anything relating to Steve, his liver and the hospital unnerves me.

I clear my throat and say, "Hello?"

"Are you Rosie?"

"Yes," I say and sit down at my desk.

"Do you have a minute?"

"Yes, of course."

After repeating her name and position, she says, "I'm responding to the complaints you made to Dan about your evaluation week at the hospital. I'd like to talk with you about that, if you have time."

I take a deep breath and say, "Of course. I appreciate your concern." I launch into my litany of complaints and then pause. "You know what, it might be better if I write this all up and send it to you. Would that work?" I learned long ago in my positions in senior management for both in-patient and out-patient physical medicine and rehabilitation centers the value of documentation.

In addition to managing all the therapy services—physical, occupational and speech therapy, social work and neuropsychology—I was responsible for ensuring that all licensing and accreditation requirements were met. Documentation was King. Surveyors from the Joint Commission for Hospital Accreditation, Medicare, Medi-Cal and the Commission on the Accreditation of Rehabilitations Facilities routinely scoured the center's medical records for evidence of compliance with their standards. The financial health of the institution depended upon the centers passing their surveys.

"Yes, that would be very helpful."

"OK. I'll send it right away." Thanks to the voluminous emails I had sent to family and friends during our evaluation week as well as my own contemporaneous notes, I whip out a three-page letter in no time and send it as an attachment. I also send a copy to Dan to keep him in the loop.

She writes back quickly to say, "Thank you, Rosie. I will follow-up with your complaint and notify you of the outcome."

Maybe some good will come of this. Maybe management will revise their transplant coordination policies and procedures to prevent the snafus we encountered. Not every family member has a medical background and knows how things are supposed to be done in a hospital. I would hate for other patients and families to become ensnared as we have been in their web of mismanagement.

Thursday, January 22, 2015
11:00 a.m.

Sitting at my computer, Sugar on my lap, I begin my list: 1) Secure kitty caretaker for Sugar and Billy for up to six months, giving Billy his asthma pill every other day, and cleaning the litter boxes. 2) Buy six months' worth of cat food, litter and medication. 3) Ask Mary Lou to take care of our mail and pay our bills; give her my checkbook. 4) Consult with Dan about helping us to find a temporary apartment. 5) Draw up a list of what to pack and mail ahead as soon as we have an address. 6) Make a list of everything to bring with us on the plane. 7) Shop for same. 8) Ask Scott to take care of any book orders that come in while we're gone and give him the materials. Steve's linguistics text is selling well to three universities offering TESOL (Teaching English to Speakers of Other Languages) certificates. 9) Buy and set up new cell phones. 10) Order the meds we will need to cover us for at least six months.

These and a few thousand additional things to be completed before we can return to the hospital. Sugar provides the warm furry comfort I need to take the edge off my anxiety.

Sunday, February, 8, 2015

Around 7:00 p.m., waves of nausea roll through me. I vomit, then vomit again and again and again. The bathroom floor is cold and hard despite the towels Steve hands me to protect my knees. Feverish, slight cough. More vomiting. I call the Advice Nurse at our health plan who suggests I rush to the Emergency Room. Not sure if it's a flu bug or food poisoning. Since Steve is not allowed to drive, and I'm too sick, I call for an ambulance.

An old childhood scene ignites: suddenly I am ten again and at the mercy of my father. For reasons that elude me even now, my taciturn but explosive dad would holler at me and my mom whenever she needed to call our family doctor to make a house call because I was ill.

Midwesterners are nothing if not stoic. I hate asking for help, but I'm too weak to gut it out.

Two strong young men help me down the stairs and into the ambulance. I feel and look like hell. Steve tells me I look just fine and rides along with us, holding my hand. I can't locate a comfortable spot on the bed's lumpy mattress. I'm jostled by every hiccup on the damn road.

They've hooked me up to an IV and are calling the hospital to notify them of our arrival. I carefully marshal my breath so I don't throw up in the damn ambulance.

As soon as the admissions clerk completes his check of my insurance and I finish signing the papers, the Emergency Room attendants roll me into an exam room. I transfer myself to the hospital bed. I worry about Steve, don't want him to catch anything. We both need to be healthy enough to return soon for his transplant and that could be sooner than we think. The nurse's assistant rushes in and hands me an emesis basin which I promptly christen. Oh joy.

The ER is full tonight, twenty-five rooms sheltering the ill and injured, some more cranky than others. The woman next door cries out, "Let me out of here. Let me out of here!" A nurse uses her soothing voice to calm her. That works for a few minutes, but the woman's plea soon erupts anew. I know how she feels.

Bells ding. Rustles of fabric, mild squeak of crepe-soled shoes as doctors and nurses rush back and forth. Two policemen walk by, dressed in their blues, packing guns. Wonder what the bad guy or gal did to merit their attention—armed robbery? Fleeing the scene of an accident? That's probably it. As we rolled in tonight, we passed a room where lay an anguished young man with his head heavily wrapped in blood-stained bandages. Mother crying. Guard at the door.

The ER doc arrives, completes his assessment, starts an IV and sets me up with anti-nausea medication. Draws blood. Orders a CAT scan. What? I tell him I cannot be put into that tube unless I'm stoned out of my mind on Ativan. That delays the CAT scan. I am still vomiting.

Need more anti-nausea meds. Coughing has increased. I am totally fucking miserable, chilly and achy, feeling as if I've gone ten rounds with a kangaroo. Steve feels helpless. I tell him to please keep his distance. He cannot afford to catch whatever the hell this is. I vomit again. How could I possibly have any food left in my system? I'm probably spewing up all my innards.

Fuck. Fuck.

It is now 3:00 a.m. Doc asks, "How are you?"

"I've been better. When's the CAT scan?" I ask, shaking my head out of its stupor. "I'm pretty stoned right now. I think I can handle the tube. I'd like to go home."

"I'll go check." Steve is still dozing in the chair. That man can sleep anywhere.

The transport attendant finally arrives to whisk me off to Radiology. I tell Steve he should stay in the room. "I'll be fine, Honey." The Ativan keeps my claustrophobia in check. I survive the trip in and out of the dreaded tube.

Back to the ER room. Vomit again. The woman next door is still screaming, still wants out.

Steve says, "I'll call Angie later and see if she can pick us up when you're discharged."

"Thanks," I say and nod off to sleep. Ativan, my sweet friend.

The doc discharges me at 8:00 a.m. Diagnosis unclear. Might have been food poisoning, might have been a stomach flu. At any rate, I'm some better. Angie, our dear friend, very kindly shepherds us home. I crawl back to bed, still nauseated, but no longer vomiting. Bad cough and congestion, whopping aches all over.

Steve brings me a cup of warm broth when I wake up. He looks ill himself. His color is yellow-gray, his sclera is yellowish, and even with Lactulose and Xifaxan, his mentation has slowed. This will all change after his transplant, I know—I hope—but in the meantime I can't expect him to do much toward getting us ready to leave. And I'm too goddamned sick to resume my plans.

I sleep off and on, weaker than a daffodil drooping at the end of its bloom. I wonder if they feel sad, knowing they won't be up and lively again until next year, or if they're looking forward to a long nap, having brightened our lives, lo these many weeks.

I made sure to thank them on my previous walks, told them how much joy they were bringing to the neighborhood, how beautiful they were and that I looked forward to seeing them again next year.

Wednesday, February 11, 2015
10:30 a.m.

Janice calls again, asks if I have a minute to discuss results of the hospital's investigation into my complaints.

I croak, "Sure." I don't need this right now, but I can't very well put it off. I need to know that they are fixing things so that when we return we will feel safe.

Janice reads from the report. "Dr. Schafer (the surgical resident during Mr. West's trip to the Emergency Room in January) has been counseled about using heparin in a patient with a low platelet count."

"That's good," I say. "Wouldn't do to have him kill a patient, now would it?"

Probably should keep my snark under control, but I'm too sick to care. I look around for Sugar and watch her bouncing up the stairs, eager to hop onto my lap. I need all the comfort I can get right now.

Janice continues. "Regarding your complaint that your phone calls were not answered on January 14, 2015, the operator reported that Ms. Sorenson had not used the word, 'urgent.' Therefore, the clinical staff were unaware of her situation."

What? I cough and start to cry. *This again?*

I hold the receiver away and shake my head back and forth. I breathe as deeply as I dare without triggering a round of coughing, dry my eyes on my sleeve, stroke Sugar with my other hand, and hope to keep the tremor out of my voice when I say, "Excuse me, but what you said just doesn't make sense. I used the word 'urgent.' In fact, I was frantic and any idiot could have heard that in my voice. Why did she think I was talking fast, telling her about Steve's confusion which was getting worse and worse, and why in the hell wouldn't the clinic staff phone me to find out what was going on, just in case?"

I have to pause a few seconds to marshal all my resources so I can continue. Take as much of a deep breath as I dare.

"We flew all the way from California to get there, didn't know a soul, were never given information about what to do in case we had an emergency. I made three frantic calls in the afternoon and when no one called me back, I called Dan all the way out in

California to get help. And then he tells me to rush Steve to the Emergency Room.

"I only got a call from Andrea, Dr. Yilmaz's assistant, as I was on my way out the door. I had already told Dr. Yilmaz about Steve's confusion and need for Lactulose when we saw him on the first day. If he had ordered a blood test for Steve and then some Lactulose, Steve wouldn't have had a near-fatal event. What's wrong with those people?"

"I'm sorry about that, but the investigator's report states that the operator said you never used the word urgent."

"That's a damn lie and she knows it; just wants to cover her ass. I want a copy of that report so I can write up a rebuttal. You work for my health plan, aren't you supposed to be on my side?" I run my hand through my matted hair.

"I'll see what I can do."

I hang up.

Steve overhears my heated conversation. I can barely splutter out the words. "They claim I never said the word 'urgent' when I called. And that was their excuse for no one helping us. In all the notes I wrote at that time and in emails to family and friends, which I still have, I used the word 'urgent.'"

"Crap, crap, crap and their damn rabbit hole."

"Crap is right," he says. "Let's go lie down." We head off to my bedroom. I flop into bed; Steve sits beside me. I can't stop bawling.

"I did the best I could to get you help and it didn't work. What if this happens again when we go back for your transplant? What the fuck am I going to do then? Do I have to fight them every minute to keep them from killing you? I can't do this, Steve." I roll over on my side to face him.

He rests his hand on my shoulder and tells me to sleep.

"Everything will be fine. Dan said the surgeons are great, remember?" He's all kindness and heart.

What do you know?

Steve is very sweet and supportive, but for all intents and purposes he wasn't "there" when this all went down. His severe encephalopathy interfered with his ability to understand what was happening.

"And, if it's not fine, then what? What am I going to say to your family? 'Uh, sorry to tell you, but I couldn't keep the hospital from killing Steve. My bad.' And what if by complaining I have interfered with your listing? What if they delay giving you a liver because of me?"

Steve often criticizes me for catastrophizing. Well, that was my job for many years—to think ahead to the worst scenarios, then plan mitigation strategies. I'm damn good at that, but I never expected I'd have to do it here, not at a well respected hospital where surgeons perform many, many transplants a year. It's exhausting.

★★★

I'm the person in whose company you wish to be when there's an emergency. I'm the one you want to sit next to on a plane when it's hijacked by terrorists. Due to my chaotic childhood, I became a vigilant adult. I'm constantly squirreling away bits of information about how to deal with scary events.

A mid-flight attack, for instance.

Here are some helpful tips: 1) Keep a sock filled with quarters in your carry-on bag. You can ease it through security, and if the need arises later, you can hit a terrorist in the head with it and drive him to his knees.

2) Roll up an in-flight magazine, nice and tight, then shove it into the offender's solar plexus. That'll make him wish he'd stayed home and watched *American Idol.*

3) I've come up with a third method, which I haven't yet had a chance to try out, but it goes like this: Remove your clothes and walk naked down the aisle toward the terrorists, while at the same time singing "Oh Beautiful for Spacious Skies." Since it's easier to sing than "The Star Spangled Banner," others will be more encouraged to chime in.

The terrorists will be so stunned by this unusual display of patriotism that they will be easily overcome by passengers wielding rolled-up magazines and socks full of quarters.

You'll thank me later.

Chapter Eight

WHAT NOW?

Sunday, February 15, 2015
11:00 a.m. at home in the Bay Area

T he phone rings. I set the newspaper aside on the sofa and head toward the office. It's Ava, transplant coordinator for the hospital, asking for Steve.

"Just a minute," I say and holler for him. He slow walks the hallway, buttoning his shirt as he goes. I stay close. They chat for a minute. I hear Steve saying, "Really? Well, that sounds good, thanks for calling; we'll let you know," and then he hangs up, a wide smile crinkling his face.

"What?" I say, my voice still raspy.

He turns to me and says, "She said, 'Where are you? We've been transplanting patients at a MELD of 19 with your blood type!' They want me there right away! We've got to get going!" He gives me a look and says, "We gotta go!"

I suck in my breath, fighting a cough.

Oh, hell. How am I supposed to pull this off?

"That's just great, Steve," and steady myself against his desk, "but there's no way I'm going to be ready for at least another week or longer. I'm still coughing, still weak, still have tons of stuff to do—" I turn away toward the bedroom.

"But they want me now!" he says and follows me, his eyes drilling my back.

"I get that, Steve," I say and flop down on the bed. "I heard you, but *now* is not going to happen." I throw up my hands, fresh out of patience. "I can't possibly move any faster than I've been moving. Why don't you call Landon and see if he can fly up here and take you? That way, I can recover, finish up with everything and then join you."

"Good idea," he says. His son lives in Los Angeles, just a quick flight up to San Francisco.

Oh, crap, shit. Fucking liver. Steve needs to fly now. Four years we've been waiting for this, and now I'm so exhausted that I've barely been up an entire day for over a week? I can't just click my heels and fly away with him. He has no idea of all the work I have done and have yet to do to arrange our absence for as long as six months, and I'm doing this on less than half of my usual energy. I feel like shit. I know he needs me, but there's nothing I can do to pull a rabbit out of this fucking hat. Nothing. I hate him.

I know he's not well and that we're lucky he's still alive and has a chance at a full life with a new liver, but this liver show has been going on for the past four years, worse during the last two. Red alert most every day. How is his ascites? How are the petechiae. How is his temperature? How is his mentation? Does he need more Lactulose? Xifaxan?

Rushing him to the ER every two-three weeks whenever his temp would rise to 100.4. Infection alert. Now—generalized sepsis and the need for powerful IV antibiotics. Now—an infection on his mitral valve, more antibiotics. Visiting him in the hospital all day, every day. Helping him at home with his meds, although I had to draw the line at taking charge of his PICC (peripherally inserted central catheter).

During one of his hospitalizations I stared at the fluoroscopy screen while the nurse inserted the flexible tube into a vein in his upper arm and then slid it up and over until it reached the outside of his heart where powerful antibiotics would be sent to the rescue. I gasped, thinking of all the ways this could have gone sideways.

Before his discharge, the nurse told me I was the one who would take care of administering his antibiotics every day through the line, and that she would show me how.

Just thinking about it made me feel faint.

"No. I can't do that," I said and backed away. "Can't I bring him to the out-patient clinic and have the nurses do it there? I'm happy to do that."

"No. You have to do this at home," she said in the way nurses have of telling you they're pissed, but without actually saying so. You just know she's thinking, *lazy bitch coward.*

I felt a scream working its way up from my diaphragm, *You have no idea what I've already been through with Steve. I'm not a fucking nurse,* but I choked it back.

No," I said. "I couldn't live with myself if somehow I screwed it up." I looked over at Steve and blew my nose, damn allergies.

"All right," she said, giving up the battle with this obviously intransigent woman (me), and turned to Steve. "Mr. West, do you think you can do this if I teach you how?" This was no idle question, more like a command from Nurse Ratched.

"Sure," he said, with full confidence. I watched him fumble at first, but she was remarkably patient, and on the third try he succeeded.

On the way home, driving, I apologized to Steve. "I'm so sorry, Honey, but I could never forgive myself if I screwed this up for you. Makes me sick just to think about it." I don't dare cry while I'm driving. The freeway buzzes with crazy drivers.

"No problem," he said. "I've got this." *Oh, Lordy, let's hope so.*

The pharmacy delivered all the materials to our home. Steve set himself up on the sofa, with a table nearby.

I stood by to hand him items, as he carefully worked through all the steps:

Washing his hands with soap and water for 40-60 seconds and drying them with paper towels; injecting saline in the tube to flush it; removing air from the syringe; scrubbing the end of the PCC line with alcohol pad for 15 seconds; twisting the syringe onto the IV line; attaching the antibiotic syringe and pushing the IV medication in slowly over 3-5 minutes; flushing the line again. I watch, amazed, that he is so comfortable performing this ritual. Twice a day. Without these powerful antibiotics, he would die. He's fortunate that the Ertapenem, the Superman of antibiotics, is working. I'm not even sure there was a back-up plan.

One evening, Steve called to me for help when his line becomes tangled. Said it was too long or something, and would I please take some scissors and "cut here" as he held out the tube? I did.

We realized too late the mistake we just made.

Off to the ER. When the Admissions clerk asked the reason for our visit this evening, I piped up and said, "Patient fucked up." That brought the only laugh of the evening. Two nurses very deftly changed the tubes, no harm, no foul, and sent us home.

Landon is unable to take time off work to fly with Steve to the hospital. Now it's all down to me.

After a few more days, I tell Steve I think I'm finally on the upswing and that we should talk to Dan, our coordinator, to set a date for our return. We check the calendar and decide that Tuesday, March 10, would work. That would still give me more time for my stamina to improve and for me to complete the thousand and one tasks on my list before we depart.

I leave a message for Dan, asking him if he could check with the hospital to find out if our travel plan would work for them. I also ask him if he can help me find an apartment. We can't manage without his assistance.

He calls back right away. "I contacted the transplant team and they're fine with you arriving on the 10th. The clock is ticking! They're eager to get Steve transplanted. I've also contacted a corporate housing company to work with you on the apartment hunt. Several of our patients have had good luck with them. They will be contacting you with some options."

"Great. You're a peach. Thanks!"

Monday, February 23, 2015
1:30 p.m.

Phone call from Cheryl Canning, Quality Assurance from our health plan.

Ms. Canning reviewed with me the hospital's report about my complaints. I didn't think to ask her why she bothered calling since Ms. Olsen had already explained the report to me over the phone.

Once again, the blame was assigned to me. If only I had said the magic word "urgent" when I made my calls, someone from the clinic staff would have gotten back to me right away.

"Wait a minute," I said, getting more and more pissed. "When I called the operator, I remember hearing a message informing callers that their call was going to be recorded for quality purposes. Has anyone listened to my calls?"

"The operator said there were no recordings of your calls."

"Of course there weren't. She's lying."

No wonder they didn't believe me.

By now I'm all out of fight and just want to get off the damn phone. I dribble out a weak statement, "This is not true. I did too use the word 'urgent.' Your operator lied. I want a copy of the investigator's report. I need to rebut this."

She said she doubted the hospital would give me a copy, but said the transplant team wanted to meet with me on March 11, the day after we arrive.

Not thinking, I said "OK. How about 1:00 p.m.?" just to get her off the fucking phone.

"Fine." Said she would schedule that and confirm it with me later.

I quickly review in my mind everything that had transpired during and after the evaluation week and smelled a rat. In my previous life, I'd seen firsthand how a hospital might deal with fear. Red alert. Circle the wagons.

Although the meeting was being scheduled ostensibly in the spirit of cooperation, I believed they were planning to confront me with a tag team of hospital defenders. To calm the little woman down.

Why the fuck would I want to walk into that?

I call her back, leave a message, saying I wouldn't attend the meeting unless I had the report in hand.

Two hours later, I receive a phone call from yet another person, this one named Candace Adams in Patient Relations at the hospital. Ms. Adams says she was contacted by Ms. Canning who told her she didn't think she could get me the report before the meeting but that the staff really wanted to meet with me.

"No," I say. "I have no desire to meet with the team without having seen the report. I don't see why there's such a problem giving that to me. There are clearly some mistakes in it, and I would like to correct the record."

"The hospital attorney won't allow you to have a copy." She says this so matter-of-factly that I wonder how many other times she'd had this conversation.

"Well, then, I see no reason to meet with any of you," I say, hang up and sigh.

★★★

Crap. What if I've just made a big mistake? I've never done this before—taken care of someone so medically fragile and having to manage alone. Aren't you supposed to be able to trust in the people whose job it is to take care of him?

It will be several years before I learn about the true extent of hospital errors in the U.S., spurred on by the consolidation of hospitals at the hands private equity companies who cut costs and increase their profits by squeezing physicians and nurses to do more and more with less and less, thereby endangering everyone.

I'm quickly learning on my own, the hard way, what patients and family members can and must do to protect themselves.

But right now, all I know is that I'm alone in this endeavor. I hope to God I can draw upon what medical knowledge I have and can summon the courage and grit I will need to see us through.

Otherwise . . .

Chapter Nine

ON A WING AND A PRAYER

Tuesday, March 10, 2015

T his is it. The day we're flying 2,000 miles again on the wings of United from California to the out of state hospital where—the "good Lord willing and the crick don't rise"—Steve will get a new liver, a new life and in a few months a safe return home.

We threw the dice—a game of liver craps, if you will—betting Steve would get a liver in this hospital well before he could ever rise to #1 on the list in San Francisco. There he would have been certain to die before his number came up.

So this is it. All or nothing, baby. I either bring Steve home with his new liver, or tuck a small cedar box containing his ashes inside my carry-on.

No pressure.

San Francisco Airport
10:00 a.m.

After we've boarded our flight from San Francisco to Denver in the cool California breeze, the pilot announces that we have been delayed by stormy weather ahead of us. He assures us that passengers will make it to Denver on time for their connecting flights. I hate having to change planes, especially with Steve, whose abdomen now is even more amplified than on our previous trip. Hurrying is no longer in our vocabulary. Nonstop flights to our destination, however, are scarce as hen's teeth, unless we want to fly the red-eye, which we do not.

We buckle up and finally take off.

"This is it, Honey," I say to a bleary-eyed Steve. "The big kahuna."

Steve puts his hand to his mouth, snorts and says, "Don't make me laugh."

"Sorry about that. I just can't take this all-seriousness-all-the-time, which I know it is—your getting a transplant and all, but still . . ." I lean in and kiss him on the cheek.

"I agree," he says, pats my hand and starts dozing.

Finally. On our way. God, I'm tired of this and I know Steve is too. If we're very, very lucky, the next time we fly, it will be with his new liver.

What could possibly go wrong?

As we near Denver and begin our descent, the pilot announces that we were not able to make up the time we lost and, unfortunately, some passengers might miss their connecting flights.

What? No, oh no, no, no, no. This cannot be. I look around and wave to the short brunette flight attendant who hurries over to us. Her name tag reads "Becky."

"Becky, we have a problem," I say, struggling to stay calm. I do *not* want to dissolve into an inarticulate mess. "We can't miss our next flight. Steve is very ill, and we're on our way to get him a liver transplant. We have to get there today." No telling when we might actually get the call notifying us they have a liver for him, but the thought of being stranded in Denver, well, that just can't happen.

Becky appears to be listening to what I'm saying, so I continue. "When we land, could you please ask the other passengers to let us off first because of a medical emergency?" She frowns and hesitates.

"Please, Becky. His life depends on him getting there in time. What if this were your dad?" I'm about to lose it. Steve looks off in the distance.

"Let me go check," she says. I slump back in my seat. What's to check? This man is dying. We can't stay all day or night in the Denver airport while we wait for another flight. We told the hospital we'd be in town on the 10th. We have to make it.

She returns in a few minutes and says, yes, she will make the announcement, but she can't guarantee that the other passengers will go along with it.

Why the hell wouldn't they? Have we lost all heart in this country?

"Thanks," I say, my mouth dry.

On the PA system, Becky announces, "We're going to land soon here in Denver. We have an emergency request for you to allow a man and his wife to leave the plane first, due to a medical issue so they can absolutely make their next connection. Thank you."

The plane touches down and Becky scurries to our row to help offload our bags from the overhead bins. When the plane finally stops, I lend Steve a hand as he scoots out of his seat and positions himself behind me with his bag.

We commence our exit, hoping the others will give us a wide berth. I'm full-out crying now and through my tears, I splutter a heartfelt thank-you to each passenger as we squeeze through the gauntlet.

"Thank you, thank you so much. I'm sorry about this. My husband is very sick and we're flying to get him a new liver, and we can't miss our next flight." Most of the passengers seem genuinely sympathetic, a few not so much. I keep crying, snuffling, wanting to crawl into a hole and die. This is too much. Steve shuffles behind me.

We finally deplane and scoot away from the gate, the fragrance of caramel popcorn welcoming us and the other passengers as they fan out to their destinations. We exhale and pull ourselves together, leaning against a nearby wall.

A young female passenger strolls by, smiles and says, "I hope everything works out all right." I nod and wave.

I turn to Steve to make sure he is OK and still hanging onto his bag. In my panic, I forgot to ask for transportation to the next gate. Bloody hell. We have five minutes. I do not want to frighten Steve.

"Steve," I say, wiping my eyes and touching his arm with fake calm. "We don't have much time. I know you can't hurry, so I'm going to run ahead of you and, if I can, get them to hold the plane. Does that make sense?"

He nods.

I look down the impossibly long concourse but don't emphasize the distance to Steve.

"Our gate is at the end of this concourse, so we need to run all the way down and then hang a right. The next gate will be around the corner. If I make it in time, I will talk to the gate person and ask her to hold the plane. I'll wave to you as you come down the walkway. OK?"

He nods again. I give him a hug. No time to make sure he understands. I whirl around and take off, trotting/running as fast as I can, pulling the small wheeled suitcase behind me, weaving in and out of other travelers, trying not to nick them as I scurry by.

Onto the moving walkway, trotting again. I'm already panting, having to stop, bend over and exhale, gathering my wits, but I must keep chugging. I turn around, wave to Steve. He's heading in the right direction, oh so slowly. If only I can get there in time, I can make them wait for him. Maybe. I start crying again. What if this doesn't work? No, dammit, I have to make it work. We can't miss this plane. I'd never forgive myself.

My suitcase wobbles behind me on old-fashioned rollers, not the new-fangled spinners which would have made it easier to maneuver. It tips. I stop to regulate it. Run, trot, run, trot, wobble, wobble, pant, pant, cry.

My lungs are burning, I do not want to go any further, don't think I can go any further, but I finally reach the end of the walkway, stumble off and turn into the gate. I pause, inhale a few deep breaths, hurry up to the counter and explain my problem.

"No worries," the gate attendant says, "we're holding the plane for you. Becky called ahead."

Now I'm bawling and shaking my head. Relief. Gratitude. I can barely eke out a "Thank you, thank you," as I bite my lip. I turn back to the concourse. Steve is snailing right to the end.

I dash up to him, coughing. "We're safe, Honey, we made it. They're holding the plane!"

7:30 p.m. Safe arrival at our new apartment

Our taxi driver hoists our many bags out of his trunk and rushes them through the flashing rain to the front door of our new apartment, only four miles from the hospital. The location makes the transplant surgeons very happy. We will be only fifteen minutes away whenever we get "the call," telling us they have a liver for Steve. Relief? Yes. Terror? Oh yeah.

I lift the doormat and find the keys where they are supposed to be, along with a note welcoming us and providing directions to our new mail box at the apartment complex, key included. A good omen, yes? I unlock and hold open the door for the driver who very kindly schleps all the bags and sets them in the dining area. I register very little of the disinfectant smell usually used in hotels and hospitals.

The corporate housing company that Dan recommended located this one-bedroom apartment for us. I signed us up sight unseen. No time to be picky. We asked for a sofabed in the living room for Steve. He can sleep anywhere. I need a sturdy door between us. The best part? Housekeeping services twice a month. Not having to worry about vacuuming, cleaning, carrying out garbage—a blessing.

Steve, more exhausted than a marathon runner, collapses onto the sofa bed and switches on the TV. Fluffy pillows and soft fuzzy blankets beckon in one corner. Together we pull the bed open, add the pillows and blankets, and he's ready for the night.

I devoured most of my snacks on the long flight from California and am famished. Nighttime and the forbidding drizzle have twinned to make me hesitate to go out again, but I see in the distance what looks like a purple neon light for a restaurant. Salvation? Maybe? I am way too exhausted to trudge anywhere. Damn Denver airport and its zillion-mile concourse. I'm too hungry to wait for a taxi.

"I'm going to get us some food, Steve. Let's make sure your cell phone is on while I'm gone." I tug the phone and his charger out of his carry-on, set them on the nearby desk and plug them in.

"I don't know what they might have there, but do you want me to get you a sandwich, if they have any?" I say as I reach for my coat hanging off a dining room chair. I shrug into it and fasten my fanny pack around my waist. Snatch my gloves and hat on my way out.

"No. I'll just have a Glucerna." Whenever he's watching a Warriors game, he's barely communicable. I don't blame him. Steph Curry dazzles.

I paw through one of our bags to claim a can; open it and hand it to him; he swallows it in one gulp.

"Have fun," he says, making a three-pointer across the room with his empty can. "Yes! Me and Steph."

I could have cut through the maze of apartments to reach the street, but then I wouldn't know how to find the apartment on my return; so I follow the breadcrumbs driveway back to the entrance.

I need a hot shower. I need my heating pad on my back and my ice pack on my neck. Sitting on a plane makes them very unhappy. But my need for food trumps everything. Outside the apartment door, I perform some standing arch and sways to loosen up my back muscles, some shoulder rolls for my neck and take off in Buddhist fashion, focusing on one step at a time, one breath at a time. My body screams for bed, but, no matter, I simply must eat now and stock up with something for morning.

On my trip down the deserted sidewalk to what I hope is a restaurant, wondering whether or not this is a safe neighborhood, my tired mind whirrs with plans for the next few days: obtain Steve's blood work and see his surgeon at 11:00 a.m. tomorrow to make sure Steve is in tip-top shape for the surgery. Stop by the hospital cafeteria to fetch more food to take home. Grab a taxi back to the apartment. Rent a car, check my new mail box to find out if the boxes I mailed ahead have arrived. Take a long, long, long nap. Then stash away clothes, toiletries and other things. The apartment has more closets and drawers than my California condo.

I arrive at the Oasis vegetarian restaurant just before closing and order six veggie wraps to go. Straggle home, rain or no rain, wolfing down one wrap as I go; inhaling another at the apartment and stashing the rest in the fridge. Steve has drifted off to dreamland, snoring.

I wheel my suitcases, one at a time, into the bedroom. Call the taxi company for our early-morning ride to the hospital. I open one of the suitcases, pull out my favorite black pants, jeans, sweaters, blouses jackets and give them all a shake before I hang them up in the spacious walk-in closet. Settle the suitcases in the back.

I step into the shower and cry again. This is all a bad dream. I can't believe we made it out of Denver. I don't want Steve to see or hear me. I must keep it together so I can manage whatever gets thrown at us. I love this no-drought city where you can stand under the hot shower as long as you want.

In bed, all the worries of the past few weeks flood in. You know you're strong, but are you strong enough?

There is no alternative.

★★★

It feels as if everything I've learned from the enormous effort I made as an adult to rid myself, with varying degrees of success, from the ongoing mental and physical torment from my now dead father is coalescing around this moment—the moment of my Big Final Exam: Saving Steve.

Nevertheless, I've not wallowed in self-pity. No, that's not the Midwestern, Lutheran way. You buck up; you take it like a man; you don't cry over spilt milk; what's done is done; you can't have your cake and eat it too; you turn the other cheek; you do unto others as you would have them do unto you; you don't cry or I'll give you something to cry about; and you'd better be a Nice Girl.

So, I've bucked up and gone on. I once figured out that my dad had 187,000 hours of direct influence over me while he was alive. Those hours were "hard time." As an adult, I've spent 34,000 hours in therapy, in personal growth seminars and workshops, lived at Esalen Institute in Big Sur, walked on fire with Tony Robbins, listened to every goddamned program on achievement motivation, self-hypnosis, and success strategies, read every relationship book and psychologically pumped myself up so many times I could play the emotional counterpart to Dana Carvey's Hans to Kevin Nealon's Franz on the Saturday Night Live sketch, "Ve've come to . . . pump you up."

I can do this!

What if I can't do this?

Wednesday, March 11, 2015
9:30 a.m.

We taxi to the hospital, ride the elevator to the lab for Steve's blood draw and then down again to stop at the café where we wait for his appointment with the surgeon, the café line growing longer and longer, like ants drawn to the honey pot. Hospital staff, dressed in blue or green scrubs, masks dangling from their necks; maintenance men in their sturdy gun metal gray pants, shirts and clunky suede work books; regular civilians like us, all mixing it up at the watering hole.

Steve stakes out a table while I join the line for our drinks.

I hear someone tinkling a Scott Joplin tune on the grand piano in the spacious adjoining lobby. I peek around the corner and see a teen girl playing for her parents. The huge glass vase of fresh flowers sitting atop the piano spreads fragrant cheer all around. On our previous trip here, we were treated to lots of Bach. Apparently, anyone is invited to play.

I pull up a chair across from Steve, hand over his espresso and start sucking on my iced tea through a straw. I had just bleached my teeth before we left. Don't want them stained already. One damn thing I can control. No telling when I will be able to bleach again.

I say, "How are you doing, Sweetie?"

"Not great. I just want this over with," he says and sips his espresso.

"I know you do, Steve," I say with a deep sigh. "I know you do. They're going to give you a great liver and then we can go home. You'll be able to teach soon again after that."

Hell, I don't know anything of the sort.

We've read all the books about what to expect. It's possible he will be able to return to the classroom in a few months. There's nothing he enjoys more than standing before a room of adoring college students and passing on his extensive knowledge of language, specifically linguistics. Steve has tons of words at his disposal, some in Turkish, others in Greek, German and Spanish, just not many of them related to feelings. But, get him talking about the Great Vowel Shift of 1400 to 1600 CE and watch out.

I'm sleuthing for tip-offs, especially now when he doesn't feel well. I know from his body language when he's stressed or happy or pissed. And from what he does and does not say. So when I ask him how he's doing, I have to sift through his answers or non-answers for clues. Does he look at me when he speaks, if he speaks? Or does he just grunt and look away? Does he respond with irritation if I ask the same question more than once? He's holding on tight. If our roles were reversed, I'd be a flaming mess.

At 11:00 a.m., we meet with Dr, Anthony, the transplant surgeon, who tells us that Steve's all-important MELD score has risen from 19 to 21. We didn't need the update to tell us his condition had deteriorated in the eight weeks since his evaluation. Our return to the hospital has been just in time. Dr. Anthony explains the entire transplant process again. This time, I'm able to take in more information than I could during the eval week. When he describes initiating "the cut" from one side of Steve's abdomen to the other, I squirm.

I'm not good with blood.

Next, we meet with Rebecca, a middle-aged nurse practitioner, who reviews a sturdy three-ring binder of information with us: the procedure, the ICU, the drugs, the blood tests, the recovery, possible complications, the things to avoid and, most importantly, the phone numbers of the transplant coordinators who are on call 24/7.

Perhaps they learned their lesson from the hot mess they made of our evaluation week.

My reaction under duress is to squirrel away these nuggets of information, just in case. Steve looks away, happy to turn over his life to me. In his defense, he's ill and overwhelmed; how could he be otherwise?

Next, off to the cafeteria to lay in some supplies until we can rent a car for grocery shopping.

We return from the hospital, flush with takeout from the cafeteria. I can't wait to return to Whole Foods, which was a life saver during our eval week. If we run out of hospital food before we can get more groceries, there's always the aptly-named Oasis.

I slip back into bed. Few people know that there's an Eleventh Commandment: "Thou shalt not stint on sleep." What do you think Jesus was doing during those 40 days in the desert?

Steve is enamored of the big-screen TV, but keeps the volume low.

8:30 p.m. Phone rings

"Hello?" I say.

"Hi. This is Susan James, one of the transplant coordinators. I'm calling to find out if Steve would be willing to be a backup for surgery tomorrow morning."

"Uh. Oh." Deep breath. "Right. Let me go check with Steve. Can you hang on a minute?"

Oh, shit. We had been looking forward to a quiet, restful day, but rest is not why we're here.

The nurse practitioner had just this morning explained the back-up process. It goes like this: the procurement committee meets whenever a new organ is available and is on its way to the hospital. Gods of Life. They decide who the lucky winner is. If a particular patient is qualified, but has some medical issues that might interfere with the surgery, they line up a back-up candidate, just in case.

No sense letting a perfectly good liver go to waste.

I race to the living room waving my cell phone. Breathless, I say, "Steve, the transplant coordinator is on the line, wants to know if you'd be a back-up for surgery tomorrow. What shall I tell her?"

"Hell, yes!" Big smile.

"Yes, Mary, he's happy to be a backup. What do we do?" I am staring wide-eyed at Steve.

"You have to be ready in the morning to come when we call. The patient is scheduled for 10:00 a.m., but the gentleman has some medical issues and might not be the best candidate. If he doesn't work out, then Steve will get the liver."

"OK."

"You have to stick around home. When we call, you will have to be here within thirty minutes. Tell Steve not to eat anything after 10:00 p.m. tonight. He can drink a little water with his morning pills."

"Right. Where do we go?" I'm starting to hyperventilate. Must calm down.

"You will go to the ER and tell them you're a back-up for a transplant. They will notify us when you arrive."

"OK. Thanks," I hang up; can feel my eyes bugging out.

I turn to Steve and explain everything, to remain calm. "Oh, crap crap crap. This could be it!" I say snuffling and hugging Steve. We've waited so damn long. It doesn't seem real.

We are very grateful for even the possibility, but sad for the family whose loved one just lost his or her life.

But—oh, no—we have no fucking transportation! How are we going to get there within thirty minutes after they call? I knew we couldn't count on a taxi; they'd been late each time we called. I do not say this to Steve. He's back with his TV.

OK, OK, OK, I say to myself as I pace around the apartment. *Think, Rosie. Think, dammit.* It's 9:00 p.m. I have to come up with something before tomorrow! I can't just tell them, "Uh, sorry, but we couldn't find a ride, but thanks for asking." How lame would that be? We fly all the way from California to get a liver and then can't get a ride? That can't happen.

I sit down at the computer, Googling for transportation possibilities. Maybe a limousine? I call a limo company. No. Maybe Enterprise Rent-a-Car. I ask if they can maybe deliver us a car tonight? No. Bus? No. Ambulance? No.

Frantic, I call Susan and say I don't know how we can get there within thirty minutes since we don't have a car yet. She says she'll check with a nearby hotel to see if they have room. We could go there tonight, check in, and be ready for the call tomorrow morning.

She calls back within fifteen minutes. No room at the inn. Then she says, "Why don't you just come to the hospital very early tomorrow morning and wait?"

"Brilliant," I say. "We will do that." I tell Steve the plan. He nods.

I call the taxi company, ask for someone to pick us up at 5:00 a.m., leaving plenty of time for them to be late, yet with time for us to still arrive early at the hospital.

I start packing, stuffing anything we might need into my carry on, including all of Steve's identification material, snacks for me—a veggie wrap, crackers slathered with almond butter, cashews, bottle of iced tea that I'd picked up from the cafeteria—my cervical bed pillow and medications, a Jack Reacher novel, fleece jacket and anything else I can think of.

Thursday, March 12, 2015

Jump up at 3:00 a.m. Dress in my clean black sweat pants and white sweatshirt with a photo of our cats, Sugar and Billy, on it. Call the taxi company, just to make sure they will send someone at 5:00 a.m. Rouse Steve at 4:15, help him get dressed.

5:30 a.m. Taxi arrives.

I guide Steve out the door and into the taxi. Return for my carry-on. Off we go. Catch my breath.

"This might be it, Steve. Wouldn't that be great? We could be home in a month with you and your new liver. Oh my God, I can't believe it." He's still groggy and just grunts. I scoot back in my seat and close my eyes, follow my breath. Need to calm down.

My phone rings. "That's odd. Who would call us at this hour?" I didn't recognize the number, but thinking it might be someone from California, I pick up.

"Hello," I say. It's Susan again. She tells me they have another possibility for Steve. He wouldn't be a backup this time, but could immediately receive a high-risk liver from a 21-year-old man who had died in a car crash. The young man had used IV drugs in the past 12 months, thus the high-risk status. She told me that their testing is so refined they could determine if he had HIV or Hepatitis C. He did not. I relay the info to Steve. We look at each other and shake our heads. We've been told that we might receive such an offer for a high-risk liver but that we could turn it down without endangering his listing status. We've also been told he's near the top of the list. They can't tell us his position exactly because it all depends on the condition of the patients ahead of him.

My God, it's raining livers.

"Thanks for thinking of us, Susan, but we're going to decline this one." I tell her we are on our way to the hospital. If Steve had been much, much sicker, we might have accepted any liver, even this one, but he wasn't there quite yet.

Then, of course, as soon as I've told her "no," worry sets in—did we just make a stupid decision, did we just blow his one chance to get a liver before he gets much closer to death?

Hells bells. This liver business ain't for sissies.

"That's fine. See you soon," she says.

We arrive at the Emergency Room by 5:45 a.m. Check in at the admissions desk. I scan the waiting room and spy a nest of chairs near the back wall. I wheel Steve over there, set his brake and start arranging the chairs so I can lie down.

If I were a drinker, this would for sure be a many-martini day.

Chapter Ten

HOLY CRAP ON A CRACKER

Thursday, March 12, 2015

The hospital releases us around 1:30 p.m., after the surgeons declare the primary candidate to be in good enough condition for a new liver. We're let down, yet relieved.

I had hoped to be more organized at the apartment and with a rental car in hand before the big event. We shop at the cafeteria for more take-out, especially hard-boiled eggs and bananas, two faves. I call a cab; we ride home in silence, exhausted from a seven-hour wait in the Emergency Room and looking forward to a long nap. Mary, the transplant coordinator, has told us that only about twenty percent of back-ups get the liver. It's still worth pursuing, though. Anything to put this liver horror show behind us.

We arrive at our apartment to find a brownish fluffy green-eyed kitty lying on our door mat, gazing up at us expectantly.

"Well, hello, Sweet Pea," I say, bending down to pet her or him. "What are you up to?"

The kitty answers with a long loud purr.

"He's pretty cute," Steve says. "Shall we invite him in?"

"Uh, I don't think that's a good idea. I mean, I'd love to, but what if he has fleas? We can't take a chance on an infestation."

"You're right," he says. "That would not be good."

"He's probably somebody's pet, just on a walkabout." I reach over and insert the key into the lock. The kitty scoots away. "See you later, kitty."

Steve says, "I miss Sugar and Billy," as we walk inside.

"Me, too." I say. "By the way, I called Sharon while we were waiting to hear about the transplant. She said the kitties are doing well and that Billy is being a good boy and taking his pill." Sharon is the vet tech we hired to look after the kitties while we were away. Billy has asthma and must have half a prednisolone tablet every other day. I'm relieved he's cooperating with her. Sugar, more high strung, has been chewing up the carpet. Poor worried babies. They're used to Mommy and Daddy being around all the time, indulging their every whim.

We met Sugar and Billy when they were dumped at the colony of homeless cat. I'm unforgiving of folks who dump their animals, but these kitties were lucky to have landed at our lake park where there are plenty of mice and gophers, as well as two-legged food dispensers to feed them and provide medical care when needed.

Billy, the strawberry blond, and Sugar, our Siamese mix, are the second and third kitties we've adopted from the colony.

Years before I met Steve, I fell in love with a hunky black panther of a cat at the colony. Right away I noticed he had a certain presence that none of the other cats could ignore. I watched as Sonny Gray and Green Eyes deferred to him, imitating his every move. If he lay down in the ditch and rolled onto his back, the others would look on as if to say, "Oh, so we're doing the ditch-rolling thing now, are we?" Then they'd perform the same maneuver. I remember the day I cautiously approached him. He gazed up at me through those intense green eyes and allowed me to stroke his silky face.

I named him Turtleman. A week prior, my neighbor's box turtle had escaped its outdoor cage, and I caught him/her throwing himself down one cement step at time from the second floor, hell bent for freedom. Struck by his bravery and by-God determination to escape, the name Turtleman, just popped into my head, and thereafter anyone who demonstrated a similar level of bravery became a Turtleman.

Shortly after my own kitty Muffin died of lymphoma, I decided to bring T-Man into my home. I had been routinely cuddling him on my walks, and on the day I proposed, he laid his head on my shoulder and sighed.

On my second date with Steve, I asked if he would drive me to the park and help me tuck the chunky Turtleman into the carrier and escort him home. Steve was smitten-worthy, but I needed to give him the "cat" test before I could become serious. Did he like cats? Would he think I was a crazy cat lady and not want to see me again?

Yes, he liked cats, and no, he didn't think I was crazy. Another test passed.

Turtleman was our beloved kitty for 16 years. When he eventually died of squamous cell carcinoma, we brought home Sugar and Billy, who had developed a sweet friendship at the park.

We did not want to break them up.

Steve and I spend the rest of our day unpacking, calling and emailing family and friends, napping and watching TV. A relief to get lost in the goings on of Brenda Lee Johnson in *The Closer*; she always nails the perp.

Wouldn't it be nice if in real life the bad guys always got their comeuppance?

Friday, March 13, 2015

Sleeping in late, gobbling a quick but hearty breakfast of hospital fare we'd brought in earlier—scrambled eggs and sausage warmed up in the embrace of microwaves.

While Steve channel-surfs in the living room, I work on my laptop at the desk in my bedroom, searching for the best price on a car rental. I scour the websites of Hertz, Enterprise, Dollar Rental, Avis, Budget and Alamo. I need to rent for at least four months, maybe longer, but there are no discounts on their sites for long-term rentals.

I turn to Priceline.com. Surely, William Shatner, its TV pitchman, will have a star deal for us. I submit a low bid on a four-month rental. Bingo! William is in a benevolent mood today. He's giving us half the rate of the other rental companies. The closest rental place for pick up is fifteen miles away.

It is too late in the day to maneuver through the commute traffic in this unfamiliar city, so I make an appointment for Saturday, 11:30 a.m. Finally, we can visit Whole Foods and bring back a ton of food for the next several days. Who knows when I'll be able to shop again? I have to carry many snacks with me at all times—hard-boiled eggs, nuts, crackers, carrots, iced tea, chocolate to keep my energy up. As I learned during the evaluation week in January, there's often little time to run to the cafeteria.

I strut to the living room to broadcast my good news. The savvy shopper! Steve has fallen asleep on the sofa, watching a rerun of *Law and Order*. He loves Mariska. I turn down the volume and leave him. Poor guy. Can't imagine what it's like to live inside his skin, knowing that death lurks at every moment, especially at those times when even well-meaning people slip up.

You will live, dammit. You have to, Steve. You do not have my permission to die, you hear me?

If I busy my mind, I can keep the existential dread from exploding out of my dissociation lock box. Of course he will be fine.

I return to my bedroom, compose some emails, make notes about our miserable experiences to date, thinking I might want to write about this some day. I also scan the *New York Times* for the news. There must be something happening in the world other than our quest for a liver:

Ukraine: Villagers Say They Saw Missile Just Before Civilian Jet Was Shot Down. The Malaysian jetliner was apparently downed by pro-Russian rebels in the Ukrainian village of Chervonyi Zhovten. Russia, of course, denies it.

Jurors Hear Harrowing Account of Boston Bombers' Hostage

In New Hampshire, Clinton Backers Buckle Up

Obama Discusses Ferguson With Jimmy Kimmel

Ever thus. Haven't missed a thing.

Saturday, March 14, 2015

I call a taxi to take us to the rental car establishment downtown. It's a clear, crisp cloudless day. We arrive at 11:30 a.m. as scheduled to find a long line of folks ahead of us. St. Patrick's Day revelers. I never knew there so many shades of green. I guide

Steve to a chair in the waiting room and take my place in line. I'm becoming a professional line stander-inner.

I hand the reservation agent the paperwork I printed out from Mr. Shatner and Priceline. The short redhead with a Southern accent examines it and says, "Well, we have one car left, a green Kia Soul," the one car in the universe that I abhor and cannot imagine living with for four months or longer.

"Uh, well," I say. "Are you sure you don't have anything else? These folks are all dressed in green—perhaps one of them would like it." I'm probably being too picky, but, truly, I hate the green Soul.

"Let me swing around back to see if anything has been turned in during the last half hour," she says and scoots out the door.

I tell Steve what I've done.

"I agree," he says. "I hate those cars."

The young woman returns and says, "You're in luck. A white Kia Rio just got turned in. Would that work?"

"Sure," I say. "That sounds fine." I have no idea what it looks like, other than it isn't green.

I sign all the paperwork, let her swipe my credit card for the deposit, say "thanks," and hustle Steve out the side door to await our trusty steed.

The young man named Jeff pulls up in our spunky-looking Kia, sets the brake and turns off the ignition. He hands me the keys and says, "Have fun."

I slide into the passenger seat, push it back as far as it will go to accommodate Steve, then climb out and assist Steve, all 230 pounds of muscle, bone and abdominal fluid into the seat.

"Is this going to be OK for you?"

"It's fine. I won't be sitting in it much anyway." He wriggles back into the seat and fastens his seatbelt.

Off we go to Whole Foods where I shop for groceries while Steve waits in the car. I return with five bags, stuffed with cat food and treats for our new kitty friend Fluffy, food for us and two six-packs of Clausthaler non-alcoholic beer. I love the taste of beer, just not the alcohol.

Saturday, March 14, 2015
4:00 p.m.

We stash away the groceries and are looking forward to a quiet dinner when the phone rings. Mary, again. Another opportunity to be a back-up. This time we'd have to stay overnight at the hospital. Could we be there in thirty minutes?

"Sure," I say without consulting Steve. I can tell he's become numb to the process, and very happy to let me take charge.

We've already been through the drill. This time we're ready. I pack some snacks in a plastic bag, grab for my carry-on and we head out the door. Arrival time, ten minutes ahead of schedule.

Mary, dressed in blue scrubs adorned with colorful birds, meets us in the Emergency Room and leads us to the second-floor transplant unit, which we know well from our evaluation week. She leads us to his room.

"The tech will come in and draw your blood in a few minutes, but in the meantime, Mr. Steve, please put on this gown." She hands it to him and leaves. He hands it to me. I hold it out as he slips into it. I carefully tie both ties in the front, and he slumps his big body into bed. I hang up his clothes in the tiny closet.

The window seat pulls out to make a bed for me. I plan to sleep in my sweats. We might not be here for very long, if the transplant works out soon for the other patient.

Steve swigs down his sleeping medication and is out and snoring before I can lay claim to my earplugs. I toss and turn on the unforgiving window seat pull-out bed, try to sleep, but check my watch every 15 minutes. Vigilance is my middle name, the gift that survives long after childhood.

The surgery isn't scheduled to start until 11:30 p.m. Don't know when Steve might get the call if that candidate doesn't work out.

Sunday, March 15, 2015
4:30 a.m.

The nurse enters our room to say that the candidate's surgery worked well and we can return home. Not wanting to drive around in the dark in an unfamiliar city, we stay until 7:30 a.m. No one seems to mind.

Arrive home about 8:00 a.m. and shuffle off to bed. At least we have a car now. Tomorrow, Monday, we plan to drive around and see a couple of museums. I call ahead to find out if the city museum still has that Benjamin West painting on exhibit featured on their website. Benjamin is Steve's seven-greats uncle who was a friend of Ben Franklin. The name Benjamin must have been in fashion at the time, much like today's Brad. This might be the last and only time we chance to see it.

Monday, March 16, 2015

Sleep in, enjoy an unstressed breakfast. Send emails and make phone calls to tell folks back home about our second backup caper.

At noon, my cell phone rings. It's Lisa, another transplant coordinator, saying she wants to speak with Steve.

Oh, my, not another back-up. I feel guilty even as I think this, but we've not had much peace and quiet since we arrived, and peace and quiet is what we need most.

Oh, well, in for a penny, in for a pound.

"Sure, I'll go get him." He's getting his snooze on in the sofa bed.

"Hey, Steve. Another call from the hospital." Steve stirs, sits up and clutches the phone. He later recounts Lisa's part of the conversation, which I cannot hear.

"Yes, this is Steve. Oh, thanks for asking. We thought we'd just drive around today, get a feel for the town and—"

"No you're not," she told him. "You will be here in 30 minutes."

"Excuse me?"

"The procurement committee met this morning—you are getting your liver today!"

Steve covers the receiver, turns to me and says, "I'm getting a liver today."

My heart flips off the high dive. What? Oh no. Holy crap on a cracker. I shift into overdrive.

"We're on our way, Lisa, thanks," Steve says matter-of-factly, as if we're driving over to pick up a pizza.

"OK, Steve this is it," I shriek. No time for hugs as I race to the bedroom. We're ready for this. We're ready for this, I say to myself. Add some things to the carry-on, back to the fridge for more snacks, while Steve gets dressed. Scoot the suitcase to the front door. Slip into my coat and hat, stash gloves in my pocket, strap on fanny pack. Suck up a deep breath, thinking I'll recall this moment for the rest of my life.

The moment before the bad things happen.

Ok. We're ready—but wait. Where are my keys? Not in my fanny pack where they're supposed to be. I race to the kitchen, check the counters, bang through cupboards, sleuth the trash, nothing. Crash down the hall into the bedroom, shuffle through my desk top, flip through the drawers, the nightstand, feeling dizzy. Industrial grade panic setting in, breathing shallow, vision narrowing. Panic is nobody's friend.

"Steve," I holler down the hall, "Do you know where my keys might be?"

"No. Where'd you leave them?" Duh. If I knew that, I'd already have them in hand, I don't say.

Ah, maybe they're in the door. I've been way distracted of late. I stumble down the hall. Jerk open the door, praying, please let there be keys. No. Slam it shut. Pivot to the living room. Not on the TV, not on the floor.

Oh my God. I've gotten Steve this far, and now I fuck up? I've been packing a lot of fear ever since we arrived, holding on tight, but, now when he needs me the most, I can't find my damn keys? Who is that stupid? What am I gonna do?

Fuck it. I'll call the police. They'll get us there in time. I'm just about to dial 911, when I return to the bathroom. There they are, my keys, hiding on the counter behind the face cream!

What a fucking idiot, I say to myself.

Take one deep breath. Don't have time for two.

Chapter Eleven

CAN'T BACK OUT NOW

"**C**ome on, Sweetheart," I say with manufactured cheer as I scurry down the hall. "This is your lucky day!"

We slow walk to the car, I help him shoehorn in, shut the door.

Spin out of the driveway, gun it down the road—first left, then two rights. Steve tells me to slow down, we don't want to get a ticket.

I refrain from telling him to stick it.

I park in the emergency parking area. Walk with Steve at the pace of a mealy bug to the Admissions desk; 27 minutes from the time of the call. I secure a wheelchair for Steve.

I glance around for an empty space in the corner. Steve is clutching our small suitcase in his lap along with one small plastic bag filled with who-knows-what. It's a big load for me to push, but push I do. We pass a fluffy-white-haired gentleman whose head is wrapped in bloody turquoise gauze, standing around in his kilt, white shirt, teal patterned suspenders and black knee socks, talking with people about how he "accidentally stepped off a curb downtown."

He failed to acknowledge the alcoholic haze of an early St. Patrick's Day celebration.

For some reason, I'm mesmerized by the man in the kilt. He wobbles over to a chair and sits next to his wife who is likely thinking, *The dumb bastard. I told him not to start drinking so early in the day, but would he listen?*

Soon, Kilt-Man's head drops to his chest, his knees flop apart and, I'm not proud of this, but I surreptitiously snap several photos of him.

Is he or is he not?

It's not as though I've never seen a penis. I once lived for a year at Esalen Institute in Big Sur where I calculate that during that time I had laid eyes on a thousand or more naked bodies, many with penises attached.

Steve sees what I'm doing and frowns. "That's not very nice," he says.

"I know," I say, sheepishly, "but it's damn funny. What else am I going to do while we wait—think of all the ways this could go wrong and I take you home in a box?"

Steve tightens his grip on the chair, his brown eyes telegraphing his displeasure. I lightly touch his arm.

"I'm sorry, but I just . . . Dr. Anthony is a terrific surgeon. He will keep you safe, I know he will." I don't know that for sure, I don't know anything for sure, but instead of crying I have to return to pretending.

"OK. No more sick jokes," I say and sit in a chair near Steve, but my eyes drift back to the man in the kilt. It looks as though he's had a nasty bump on his head. He might have a concussion or worse, and here I am laughing and taking pictures? Bad Rosie. I hope the docs can treat him soon.

I don't dare ask Steve how he's doing. He doesn't like to talk about difficult things, and there's no reason for me to push. This may be the last time I see him, and I don't want to recall the very moment I stepped over the line. I must summon my inner cheerleader to perk him up, tell him he will be fine, that he will get a fantastic new liver and we will soon go home. That's the only thing I need to do right now.

I can always check out Kilt-Man's photos later at home.

It is now 5:00 p.m. We've been sitting in the ER since 12:30 p.m. I hope they haven't forgotten us. We need to get this show on the road.

Lisa, the tall, thin blond transplant coordinator who called us at noon, rushes into the ER. I guess it's pretty obvious who the transplant patient is—Steve's huge abdomen is a dead giveaway.

"I'm so sorry," she says and extends her hand. "We can't always predict how things are going to go, but your room is ready now."

"That's fine, Lisa, we understand." She shakes Steve's hand, then mine.

We follow her to the elevator for a quiet ride, stop off at the familiar transplant floor where Steve was hospitalized in January. We follow Lisa into Steve's new room. I'm in a wooden daze; nothing's real. I am performing as a sentient adult, more from rote muscle memory than from present consciousness.

"The nurse will be here in a few minutes to help you into bed and set you up. When the surgeons are ready for you, you will be transferred to the surgical unit in this same bed. Dr. Anthony will be in shortly to review everything with you and to answer your questions. We're so glad you're getting your new liver today!"

She shakes our hands again and pushes open the door.

"This is it, Honey, your big day," I say through watery eyes and a deep breath while I'm giving him a hug. "From now on, you won't have to worry about your platelets, your big abdomen, your petechiae, your fatigue, your itching— all that will go away when your new liver kicks in. You'll have your life back. And I'll have my Steve back."

But do I believe any of this?

"About time," he says and shakes his head. "I'm sick of this."

Nurse Cathy comes in, a kindly gray-haired woman in rose-colored scrubs who introduces herself and begins her work. She transfers Steve easily to the bed, helps him out of his clothes, which she hands to me and says, "You will need to hang onto these while he's in surgery." She quickly gowns him and settles him into bed. She hooks him up with oxygen and an IV.

"You're all set," she says and nods. "Dr. Anthony will be in shortly. Good luck with everything. You're in good hands. He's the best."

I unzip our suitcase and cram his clothes into it, and push it aside with my foot.

"Well, dang!" I say. "Can you believe it? Your new liver? Today?"

Steve smiles. "I'm ready."

Dr. Anthony swings open the door and says, "Hi, Mr. West, Rosie. How are you guys doing?" He's as young and cute as ever. He pulls up a chair and begins describing the procedure which sounds exactly like farm stories Steve has told me about gutting a hog. We've heard the depiction before, but I appreciate his being thorough. "Any questions?"

"What do you know about the donor?" asks Steve.

"What I can tell you is that he was young and healthy and killed in a motorcycle accident. He was a big man like you, so his liver should be a good fit."

Hearing this, I suddenly feel green around the gills. His family must be distraught, losing their son or brother or uncle or father. What a tragedy. It doesn't feel right to be happy about this.

I look from Steve to Dr. Anthony and back again.

"How soon can I see him after the surgery?" I ask, eager to jump ahead, have the surgery and recovery behind us so I can take him home.

Little did I know.

"You'll be in the waiting room, right?" He smiles.

I nod. Brilliant teeth. Braces, maybe, when he was a kid.

"After the surgery and while Steve is in recovery, I will call you into the family room and tell you how it went. After that, Steve will be transported to the Intensive Care Unit where the nurses will need some time to get him cleaned up. When they are ready, one of them will come and get you."

"OK," I nod weakly. "Thanks."

Tuesday, March 16, 2015
11:00 p.m.

Finally, two male attendants arrive to transport Steve to the surgical unit.

"How're you doing Mr. West?" they say as they unlock the wheels on the bed and maneuver him out of the room with me trailing behind, pulling the wobbly carry-on.

They're all cheery, like we're just traveling to the water park for some fun in the sun.

Steve is drowsy but says, glancing from one to another and then to me, "I'm fine. Guess this is it, huh?"

"Yes it is, Mr. West. You're gonna be fine. These surgeons are the best."

"So we've been told," I say. "I'm Rosie, by the way. Nice to meet you."

"You, too. I'm Dave and this is Randy." Randy waves.

We're entering an episode of the Twilight Zone, everything in black and white, on our slow motion drive down the hallway.

I hear the distinctive voice of Rod Serling: "From this moment on, Rosie and Steve's companions will be terror, their route fear, their next stop—the Twilight Zone!"

We reach the entrance to the surgical unit. "This is as far as you can go, Mrs. West," Dave says and punches the button to open the doors.

I want to scream—No no, this is all a mistake, he's fine. He doesn't really need a liver. Please don't take my Honey away where I can't be with him.

The door hisses open. I lean in to kiss him and say, "You're gonna be fine, Sweetheart."

He nods. And off they go.

I must have looked a fright because the attendant Dave points to the other big door. "The waiting room is right through those doors, Mrs. West."

"Ah. So it is. Thanks." I bite my lip, pivot and push open the doors into the cavernous waiting room, dragging my carry on behind me, feeling more abandoned than a three-week-old kitten who's just lost her mom.

I stop, stand and stare, at nothing in particular and weep. I'm the only one here.

Now what?

It is nearing midnight. I try to doze on the three ottomans I've shoved together, but doze is all I can do, even with my sleeping meds. Rain begins a slow drip onto the skylight, then slamma-jamma, rattling the glass as if pelted by drumsticks.

The nurses keep me in the loop during the next few hours regarding the progress with Steve's transplant: now, injecting the happy drugs; now, the liver has arrived; now, the surgeon has made "the cut." Never have those words sounded so sinister. Too late to back out now. Damn the torpedoes and all that rot. It is out of my hands and into the hands of Dr. Anthony, the other surgeon and staff.

Another nurse comes out to tell me, "The old is out, the new is in." You hope Steve's angels have flung open their wings to provide a protective canopy because there's nothing you can do now to keep him safe. Nothing.

★★★

Now you wait.

Patience has never been your strong suit. You're being assaulted by a continuous blast of cortisol, the brain chemical that keeps you wired for fight or flight.

While short bursts can be useful to, say, escape the talons of a Pterodactyl, long, sustained bursts can damage your health. According to the Mayo Clinic, "Chronic stress puts your health at risk. When you face a perceived threat, a tiny region at the brain's base, called the hypothalamus, sets off an alarm system in the body . . . . Through nerve and hormonal signals, this system prompts the adrenal glands, found atop the kidneys, to release a surge of hormones, such as adrenaline and cortisol."

The report continues, "The long-term activation of the stress response system and too much exposure to cortisol and other stress hormones can disrupt almost all the body's processes. This puts you at higher risk of many health problems, including: anxiety, depression, digestive problems, headaches, muscle tension and pain, heart disease, heart attack, high blood pressure and stroke, sleep problems, weight gain, problems with memory and focus."[1]

In other words, stress can kill. I have no way to know now that after I survive the next three horrible, no good, very bad months (to borrow from the title of Judith Viorst's book), and return home with a successfully transplanted Steve, my body will revolt and propel me into the emergency room.

Shortly after I return home, I will take the first of many trips to the ER, with an eventual diagnosis of cyclic vomiting syndrome, aka abdominal migraine, during which I will uncontrollably toss my cookies every few weeks or so. Nasty, exhausting business, but I do finally lose those last ten pounds.

In the second year, I will land in the coronary care unit of my favorite hospital, having been diagnosed with two blocked arteries, thankfully, skillfully fixed with angioplasty and a stent. That's when I learn of the dangers to my heart of ingesting too much ibuprofen every day for years. That's also when I learn that I hate fentanyl. Gak. I'm just not meant to be a druggie.

Wednesday, March 17, 2015
9:30 a.m.

Steve's surgeon, Dr. Anthony, calls me to the family room to reassure me that the surgery has gone well and that a nurse will come to me after they've cleaned him up and will accompany me to the Intensive Care Unit where he will be recovering for at least a week.

I leave the family room a zombie, still holding tight to all my feelings. Relief and gratitude of the oceanic kind just slay me. I stumble into the bathroom to cry. Maybe I can breathe now;

maybe I can sleep. I slide over to the computer in the waiting room to email family and friends back home. Everyone has been praying for Steve.

The nurse who guides me at 1:15 p.m. from the waiting room to the ICU warns me that even though they've cleaned him up, Steve will still look pretty beat up. I prepare myself mentally by recalling how my best male friend, Grant looked in the ER soon after he died two years ago from an abdominal aortic aneurysm. The breathing tube claimed most of his beautiful mouth, but he was still Grant. And not Grant. I'd never before seen a dead body outside of a casket.

The nurse escorts me into Steve's room, my breath catches. *Must stay calm.* It's still Steve, but—tubes are snaking out of every conceivable strip of his body, some for introducing drugs, others for draining fluids, I'm told. His skin is gray, his cheeks are sunken, cadaverous.

I'm perched on the plaid vinyl window seat in Steve's warm room in the ICU. I've shoved my suitcase and other bags into the tight closet. Thirty-six hours without sleep.

Four nurses bustle around him in choreographed fashion, checking his fluids, his monitor, his bandages, talking to him as they work.

"How're you doing, Mr. West?" Eyes still closed, he nods, but can't talk because of the breathing apparatus. I know he hates that.

"Rosie is here now."

"Hi, Sweetheart, you made it!" I say. He grunts a greeting.

Blood stains everywhere. I long to lie down and nap, but I'm caught by the nurses' worry. They can't seem to get the bleeding to stop on the right side of his neck where another tube is still in play. For years before his surgery, his platelets hovered around

30,000. The normal range for an adult is 150,000 to 450,000. The surgeons had assured me that prior to operating they would pack him with platelets and whole blood before "the cut." Said they did that all the time.

More nurses stream in to work on him: now five, now six, now a surgical resident calling out for "more albumin, more platelets, more whole blood, more gauze." A nurse scurries back and forth to fetch the life-saving products.

They know I'm here, watching. What they don't know is how difficult it is for me to not scream, *Do you know what you're doing? Why don't you call in the surgeon?* I'm swaying on a razor's edge.

An old joke comes to mind: "The surgery was a success, but the patient died."

I long to relax and put my faith in his caretakers—this is, after all, a fine hospital—but even in the best of hospitals thousands of patients die every year from preventable medical errors. Steve almost joined that list when we were here in January. I am ferociously determined that Steve will *not* become a statistic.

Everything I have learned from my years in health care management and a career in psychotherapy I will put to good use during his recovery over the next few months.

Saving Steve's life seems to be my calling. What if I blow it?

★★★

The miracle of Steve's new liver would not have been possible without the dedication and expertise of the "Father of Liver Transplantation," Dr. Thomas Starzl, a surgeon on the staff of the Veterans Affairs hospital in Denver.

Dr. Starzl performed the first successful liver transplant on May 5, 1963. Although this patient died from pneumonia within a few weeks, it is still considered a successful transplant because no other previous patient had ever survived the difficult surgery.

The first of Dr. Starzl's liver transplant patients to survive more than a year took place in 1967. In addition to his long surgical career Dr. Starzl also conducted research into anti-rejection drugs, which hold the key to a patient's survival.

Dr. Starzl died in 2017 at the age of 90. Thousands of people, including Steve and I owe him a huge debt of gratitude.

In 1984, Congress passed the National Organ Transplant Act. That law created the Organ Procurement and Transplantation Network's (OPTN) board, made up of industry experts who were tasked with establishing policies regarding organ transplantation.

In addition, the United Network for Organ Sharing (UNOS) was created to carry out those policies by relying on independent organ procurement organizations to persuade families to donate their loved ones' organs, and to arrange for the organs to be removed and delivered to transplant centers.

In March of 2023, the Biden administration announced its plans to modernize the system of organ sharing in order to reduce the number of patients who die while on the wait list and to conduct research into racial inequities.

Chapter Twelve

YAY!

Wednesday, April 1, 2015

A pril Fool's Day. Not that I'm superstitious, but this is to be the day I bring Steve home to the apartment. I hope it's not some cosmic joke—payback for the two weeks of relative peace we've experienced, first in the ICU and then on the transplant unit. As the saying goes, "If you want to make God laugh, tell her your plans." We plan to return to California in a few weeks. *Ha.*

Steve's transfer from the ICU to the transplant unit has gone smoothly. The bleeding from the right side of his neck finally gave up, aided by more whole blood, platelets and plasma. His own platelets have soared to 94,000, still under the traditionally normal level. But hey, from a low of 28,000 at times, 94,000 feels as if we have won the lottery.

His intubation tube has been removed, the vocal cords rebounding so that he no longer sounds like Marlon Brando in *The Godfather.*

His initial liver enzymes were high, and the worry was that the liver might be headed into a downward spiral. The remedy?

Another liver. Or death. I hold my breath for two days until the values turn around.

His kidneys start perking up, no need for dialysis. Kidneys do not like to share territory with interlopers, i.e., new organs. They're like cats in that regard. *Who the hell do you think you are to take up residence in my home?* They hiss and shoot out their claws.

Steve needs at least 11 different meds, all designed to prevent his body from rejecting his new liver. The nurses draw blood at a minimum of once per day so the doctors can monitor particular values and then tweak his meds, if needed, to achieve the right balance. Not unlike a symphony conductor who takes the measure of the instruments as they perform. If the oboe is sounding a bit flat, the conductor might bump up the flutes; if the violins play too fast, she might adjust the tympani, all in the service of harmony and homeostasis.

During the two weeks before discharge, I attend a three-hour meeting with the transplant pharmacist, Eric, and one of the coordinators, Joanie, to learn about all the drugs Steve will need for the rest of his life. We, the caretakers, will be responsible for administering them, at least for several weeks until our loved ones are able to manage for themselves.

The mother of one of the other patients and the patient's wife also attend. Their son and husband is 25 years old and having a hell of a time right now on the drugs, exhibiting fits of rage. I've heard his outbursts. Even with the doors closed, he matches decibel for decibel the screams of a murder victim being stabbed repeatedly.

The pharmacist says the problem will resolve eventually, but that right now the young man must keep on taking the drugs to prevent rejection. God bless the nurses who care for all our broken loved ones. The mother and wife telegraph their extreme worry—sadness and fear etched in the deep creases on their faces and the quaver in their voices. No one speaks about the underlying cause of the young man's liver failure.

I don't mention my gratitude for Steve's strong constitution which allows him to accept these powerful drugs with seemingly no side effects.

So far.

The pharmacist also warns us that it is not uncommon for patients to experience a bout of rejection during the first few months. What then? Emergency hospitalization. *Is there to be no peace?* He stresses that "there can be no mistakes with these medications."

Steve takes a walk every day using his walker, guided by a nurse or a physical therapist. By the time he is discharged two weeks hence he can walk the length of one very long hallway, with guidance. That's about the same distance from the parking lot to our front door. He has also been given a home program of exercises, which he performs daily while sitting in his chair.

The swelling and discoloration in his left arm is doing the skedaddle. When I first saw him in the ICU, the arm was as bulbous and deep purple as an eggplant. Horrified, fearing gangrene, I said what the hell? The doctor ordered an ultrasound and reported there was no danger of him losing his arm, that such a reaction happens sometimes because of the IV that was placed in that location and not to worry.

Good to know.

Not all has been rosy, however. Late one evening when I wasn't with him, a couple of nurses scolded Steve for needing help so often to pee in the urinal. Lasix, a diuretic, is designed to make him pee buckets. In his case, frequent peeing is necessary to rid his body of excess fluid, especially from his swollen legs, whose skin is cracked and yellow.

What about that could they not understand?

On his own, Steve spoke to his morning nurses who made sure the other two would no longer be on his schedule. I was proud of him for that, one less thing I needed to fix. I have seen no evidence, but I worry that the shit storm of the evaluation week, including my vigorous complaints, might reverberate and poison current staff and interfere with his care. Nevertheless, I make a point of thanking each and every staff member who cares for Steve. And I mean it.

Taking care of patients can be a bitch of a job and when it's done well, it's a thing of beauty.

Steve also has developed an odd sore on his butt, apparently not a pressure sore, the bane of hospitals everywhere. A wound care specialist has examined him and ordered a special cream.

Steve has lost sixty pounds since his surgery just two weeks ago. Before the surgery, Steve could hoover up his meals in scant minutes, while I made my way slowly around the plate. Some of his meds interfere with his ability to taste anything. Also, his new large liver makes him feel full all the time. I sit with him at most meals, offering, "one more bite, one more bite, please?" His appearance is morphing into skeletal terrain, the skin on his formerly muscled legs and arms now flaccid.

He is still my honey, though, and still alive. Yes, still alive. They haven't killed him yet. Skinny or not, I love him and can barely contain my eagerness to whisk him away to California and return to our "real" life—his teaching, our kitties, our friends. I long to reclaim my own life, too, a life where I am not responsible for the very existence of another human being, where I can return to creating a second edition of my book about the homeless kitties

I have cared for these past fifteen years: *They Had Me at Meow: Tails from the Homeless Cats of Buster Hollow*. The book received terrific reviews from Best Friends Animal Society Magazine, from Ed Anser, Jeffrey Moussaieff Masson, Catherine Coulter and others. My readers were eager for an update on Buster, Girly Girl, Turtleman and the other stars of the book.

Shortly after it was published, Steve received his diagnosis of "non-alcoholic, cryptogenic, end-stage liver disease," dooming my sequel.

Before Steve's eventual diagnosis, the only suspicious hallmark was a low platelet count. At that time, he received the diagnosis of idiopathic thrombocytopenia purpura of unknown origin and underwent a painful bone marrow biopsy to suss out the source. The test yielded nothing out of the ordinary.

What with doctors' appointments, emergency hospitalizations for sepsis and other problems, I had little bandwidth left for my own projects.

When Steve's surgeon, Dr. Anthony, arrived on the transplant unit to check on him shortly after he was transferred from ICU, I asked if he had learned anything from Steve's old liver that would give us a clue as to why it failed.

"No," he replied, "Afraid not. When I went in, his old liver was so small and desiccated I initially thought it was the pancreas."

Upon hearing that, a wave of nausea rolled through me. Steve's new liver had arrived just in time.

Steve's sister, Jan Schrock, flew in from Maine several days after his surgery and has been staying with Steve at night in the hospital so I can get some rest. Jan is the wondrous sort of person whose joy infects everyone. With her shock of white hair, sparkling eyes, and eagerness to make contact, no one can resist her.

Jan is the perfect spokesperson for Heifer International, the organization their father, Dan West, an Indiana farmer and National Youth Director for the Church of the Brethren, founded in 1940. She is thoroughly comfortable talking with anyone and everyone—from Heifer's recipient families in Honduras or India to Steve's nurses and doctors—about the organization.

As she explained to anyone who would listen, the idea came to Dan during his volunteer stint with Christian World Service during the Spanish Civil War. Dan's job was to pass out rations of powdered milk to orphaned children. When the supply ran out, he suddenly realized that what they needed most was not a handout, but a reliable source of food and income—"not a cup but a cow." He returned home to his farm in Indiana and presented the idea to several Brethren congregations. One by one, three farmers stood up and each offered a dairy cow: Faith, Hope and Charity. They, along with others, were sent to Puerto Rico in 1944. Several thousand heifers soon followed to war-torn countries in the aftermath of WWII.

Since then, Dan West's simple, compassionate idea has grown into Heifer International, a non-profit organization which has served over 125 countries and lifted more than 100,000,000 people out of poverty.

Steve's nurses and doctors became a rapt audience for Jan's stories about the organization's humble beginnings and how most of the recipients of the livestock are women who receive training in animal care for a year prior to receiving their high-quality animal. With their newfound income from only one dairy cow, they can feed their families and send their children to school and in the process, they themselves learn how to read and write. When the first offspring of their animal is old enough, it is presented to another family in a "Passing on the Gift" ceremony, and the cycle begins all over again.

When she wasn't regaling the staff with stories about Heifer, Jan and Steve spent much of their time swapping old farm stories. One of Steve's favorites was the one about their backyard outhouse. Since their father frequently traveled on church business, his wife Lucille was left to care for the farm and her five children, in addition to teaching full time. Lucille, a dutiful housewife of the 50's, could nag her husband only so much about getting rid of the outhouse in the back yard.

There it stood year after year, a rebuke to her desires.

One spring when Steve was home from college, Lucille told him she'd had enough, saying, "Let's go burn it!"

They trekked to the back yard where Steve urged her to retreat to a safe distance while he splattered a one-quart Mason jar full of gasoline all over the insides of the outhouse. He stepped back 15 feet, lit a match and tossed it in.

Kablooey! That outhouse fire sent up smoke signals for miles and miles.

"Mom let out a wild-eyed shriek of joy," said Steve, "like it was the most delicious thing she'd ever seen."

"Oh my God," said Jan, laughing. "What did Dad say when he returned home and saw the wreckage?"

"Not one word."

Our days became a little less bright after Jan returned to Maine.

Chapter Thirteen

REINFORCEMENTS

Wednesday, April 1, 2015
4:00 p.m.

S erendipity. Steve's son Landon had made arrangements
several weeks ago to fly in tonight from Los Angeles before
we even knew the date of Steve's discharge. Landon's timing
couldn't have been better if he'd been a psychic able to peer into
Steve's future.

As with many hospitals, the discharge process deserves the
sobriquet, "Hurry Up and Wait." They are eager to move
patients out, but not efficient enough to pull off the discharge
as scheduled. It's as if they have mixed feelings about saying
good-bye. Stay. Go. Stay. Go. Not unlike the end of relationships
I've witnessed.

At the hospital, we wait for the medical equipment company
to deliver Steve's new walker. Eric, the pharmacist, breezes in
to make sure we're clear on all the meds and how to use them.
When I say "we," I really mean "me." Steve is not able to manage
his meds yet and won't be for a few more weeks. Eric informs us
that from now on, at the direction of our health plan, all of Steve's

prescriptions will be dispensed from a nearby Walgreens. Steve's nurse eventually hands us the schedule for Steve's follow-up appointments and blood draws.

Finally, finally, two attendants arrive to wheel Steve and all our baggage down to the car. I have parked in front of the Emergency Room entrance for easy access. They're quick as cats in transferring Steve to the passenger seat and all our belongings into the trunk. A new Olympic sport, perhaps? *And the Americans run away with the gold!* the announcer will crow. A light spring shower has settled in and along with it, intense humidity. We flip up the hoods of our rain jackets.

We arrive safely at our apartment. Steve holds onto my arm as we slowly walk to our front door. When we arrive at the apartment, Fluffy, our itinerant cat, awaits us at our front door, as if to say, *it's about time you got home. You may pet me now.* Steve slowly bends down to give her a light scritch between her ears as she leans into him and purrs.

Fluffy has been turning up every day for food and treats. If it weren't for our concern about fleas, she'd be living with us already. A neighbor told me that Fluffy, the little vagabond, wanders from apartment to apartment. That breaks my heart. Every kitty should have her own home and people to love and take good care of her.

I miss my daily walks around the lake at home to feed our gang of homeless kitties—Buster, Girly Girl, Maude, Green Eyes, Momma Gray, Blackberry and all the others. I lined up several excellent two-legged food dispensers in my absence. I speak with them frequently about the kitties. So far, everyone's doing well, though coyotes have been spotted once again at the park. I have to tuck that information away in my dissociation folder. Nothing I can do so far away from home. And, actually, there's nothing I can do at home either because coyotes are protected under California law. All we can do is work to find homes for the kitties with kind people who will whisk them away from the eager jaws of those predators.

Home sweet home, here we are. Steve jostles out of his jacket and eases onto the sofa bed and switches on the TV while I scurry around to ready things for Landon. I open up all the windows to draw in fresh sweet air from the jasmine plants on our patio.

Maintenance has brought us a rollaway bed for Landon and set it up in the dining room. They've also installed grab bars in the shower and near the toilet. I'm feeling a tad guilty about taking over the bedroom, but if I don't get adequate sleep, we're all doomed.

Housekeeping came in this morning, washed the dishes, returned them to the cupboards, vacuumed the carpets, scrubbed the counters, opened up the rollaway and made the bed. Ditto mine and Steve's, with fresh linens. Emptied the garbage. Dusted everything. Windexed the windows.

When I gaze at Steve, my now gaunt, but alive sweetheart, I realize a quick return home to California might be but a fantasy. I tease him about my plan to feed him like a goose, foie gras style, absent gavage, to regain some of the sixty pounds he has lost. He is not amused.

I shuffle off to my bedroom, fire up my laptop and send emails to everyone: "We're home at our apartment! Landon's coming! Yay!! Hope to be home in California SOOOOON."

Landon is 6'3" and strong, just what we need in case Steve should require more physical help than I can provide, which would be none. He has three children and designs refrigeration systems for grocery stores and other businesses. All in all, a fine young man. He's experienced in caring for the occasional hospitalized family member.

I shopped a few days ago at Whole Foods to make sure we have everything we and Landon might need. Also ventured into a local Walgreens to procure several cartons of Glucerna.

I ask Steve what he wants to eat, hoping he'd say pizza with all the toppings, followed by a cheeseburger and fries.

"How about a Chocolate Glucerna?" he says, eyes fixed on the TV.

"Sure." I grab a can and walk it over to him. "Anything else you'd like? I got you some of that good hamburger you like, or—"

"No, Glucerna is fine." I've no time to fuss with him about eating. He's going to need more than Glucerna to regain his weight. But, as an old friend was fond of saying, "That's a raga for another day." I cook and eat a couple of soft-boiled eggs, followed by a pear and a croissant.

7:00 p.m.

Time for a brief lie-down before Landon arrives. Steve is happily engaged with Harrison Ford in *The Witness*. I snatch my cold pack from the freezer, carry it to the bedroom and place it on my pillow for my neck and pull the heating pad out of the nightstand for my back. I did some sleuthing and located a chiropractor a few towns away who practices the same type of upper cervical chiropractic I'm used to. I don't know when or if I might have a chance to visit him. I brought a flash drive which contains my x-rays and the directions so he would know how I've been adjusted.

I set the alarm and doze for 45 minutes, mighty grateful that Landon has agreed to come for a week. Before Steve became too ill to travel, we would fly to LA a couple of times a year to be with Landon and his kids.

After my nap, I open up Steve's carry on and extract the dozen or so bottles of drugs he's required to take. I arrange them on the dining room side of the counter in alphabetical order so I can easily find them: some for rejection, some for infection, some for sleep, some for high blood pressure, some for blood sugar and others.

The voice of Eric, the transplant pharmacist, echoes, "The meds must be taken *exactly* as directed on the blue card." Oh so many ways for this to go wrong. I open each bottle of his evening meds, grasp one or two as required, and flipping into true OCD mode, review them once, twice, three, four times, staring at the list, staring at the small bowl I've placed them in to make sure I'm doing this just right. If he's going to die, I don't want it to be because I messed up.

"Do you want to take your pills with Glucerna or water?" I ask.

"Glucerna." I bring him the bowl. He upends the pills onto his palm and swallows them in one gulp—little soldiers marching toward victory. In fact, this entire transplant experience is a duel between the miracles of science and the body's natural proclivity for warding off strangers.

8:00 p.m.

Phone rings. It's Landon. His flight has just landed, and he is heading out to catch a taxi. "Great," I say. "We're not that far from the airport—should only be about 20 minutes. Call me when you arrive at the front gate. I'll walk over and direct the driver to our apartment. Otherwise, you might be driving around for a while."

I pat down my sweater and pants, brush my teeth, reapply my lipstick and head toward the living room.

"Hey, Steve, that was Landon. He'll be here in about twenty." Steve has fallen asleep with the remote in his hand. Poor baby. He deserves all the naps he can get. Living through a liver transplant is monstrous; but dying without one would have been worse.

Landon calls again, they're at the gate. I slip into my jacket and hustle through the apartment complex. The rain has slowed to a slight trickle.

"Hey there," Landon says, when he opens the taxi's back door. I scoot in beside him and give him a hug.

"Thanks so much for coming. Steve's really looking forward to seeing you."

The taxi pulls up to the keypad; I punch in the code for the gate and give the driver directions. We stop at our apartment; Landon pays the driver.

I swing open our front door. Landon steps in, sees his father and says, "Hey, Dad, how're you doing?" If he registers the changes in his father's appearance, he gives away nothing as he drops his bags near the bed.

I rush to lend a hand as Steve struggles to push off the bed to stand up, saying, "Well, hey there, Dude, I'm doing just fine. Thanks for coming!" Landon gives his Dad a big old son hug. Steve slumps back down.

"Looks like they're doing better for you this time than they did during the evaluation week," Landon says. "That sounded terrible."

"So far so good," I say and sigh. "Would you like something to eat?'

"Nah, I had some snacks on the plane. I would like to use the bathroom, though."

"End of the hall and on the left."

For the first time today, Steve smiles.

Thursday, April 2, 2015
8:00 a.m.

Landon drives us in our small Kia Rio, me folded up in the tiny backseat, Steve riding shotgun for his blood draw at 8:30 a.m.

I introduce Landon to the cordial clinic personnel. "So nice you could come visit your dad," they all say. Landon's charm and his sturdy physique do not go unnoticed by the mostly female staff.

After that, we are scheduled to meet with Nelly, one of Steve's transplant coordinators. I haven't yet figured out why there are so many coordinators, since few have more than a passing acquaintance with Steve.

"So, Nelly," I say, after we make our introductions and sit down. "Are you the main coordinator we should contact if Steve has any problems?"

"Yes, that's me," she says quickly. Her gruff, dismissive demeanor does not inspire confidence. Since we do not plan to be here for more than a couple more weeks, I guess we can deal.

"Good to know," I say and use my best Nice Girl smile. No need to offend. Nelly takes Steve's blood pressure, performs a physical exam, making a cursory examination of his abdominal sutures. "These are healing nicely. Do you have any pain?"

"No," Steve says. In fact, he's had little to no pain in his abdomen throughout this ordeal. I would have thought that if someone were to wield a staple gun and shoot 69 staples into your stomach, you might feel a twinge. But, no. He has not needed the opioids they've prescribed. I stashed them away, just in case.

He only feels twinges if he sneezes or has to sit up directly. He's learned to avoid pain by rolling over in bed and pushing himself up.

"She's interesting," Landon says after we're clear of her office.

"That's very kind, Landon," I say and sigh. "We're just trying to get by as best we can until we can go home."

We boogie on back to the apartment in time for Steve's home visits with a nurse, an occupational therapist and physical therapist, in that order, all professional, kind, caring people.

Landon and I look on throughout their exams, just a couple of parents watching their grade schooler perform for his teachers, hoping he gets all As.

Steve loves to be the center of attention and is happy to converse with anyone about anything. And whenever he can slip into professor mode and talk about the English language, so much the better. He charms everyone.

The nurse, Mary Jane, conducts a comprehensive physical exam and asks Steve some mental status questions. His brain is still a bit fuzzy from his ordeal, but he's so bright and fluent, that most would never know. She encourages Steve to eat as much as he wants, but stresses, fruits, veggies, whole grains. Right. She reviews his medication list and compares it with the one she's been given. Says she will see him again in a couple of days.

The occupational therapist, Michelle, assesses the safety of the bathroom and is impressed with the grab bars in the shower and near the toilet. She observes Steve donning and doffing his shirt, jacket and pants and makes recommendations to him about how he can do those more easily. He tries, but fails to pull on his pressure socks, even with his special device. I tell Michelle that I always help him with that. She gives Steve a few tips to make it easier for him to do it alone, but he's not strong enough yet.

The physical therapist accompanies Steve down the hall and back with his walker. Tells him he's doing really well. Watches Steve do his home exercise program, reminds him of the ones he has forgotten, and says that next week they will start walking outside.

I collect all their cards and ask them who I should call in an emergency.

Nelly.

Around 4:30, p.m., I receive a call from Nelly. "We've received the results back from Mr. West's blood tests. The doctor wants him to double up on the Prograf."

I make a note on his medication list.

During my evening dispensing of his meds, I do as I'm told.

How was I to know?

Chapter Fourteen

You Have No Idea

Good Friday, April 3, 2015
8:30 a.m.

I 'm a lapsed lutefisk Lutheran, but even I know that today is the day Jesus was arrested in the Garden of Gethsemane and later crucified.

Many lifetimes ago, I sat in the Garden of Gethsemane at the foot of an eight-hundred-year-old olive tree with a group of followers of an Indian guru from Oakland, Sant Keshavadas, as he led us in a goose-bumping meditation. His haunting, chanting voice summoned tears in everyone, even in me.

That memory was top of mind as we drove Steve for his 8:30 a.m. blood draw, only to find the Transplant Clinic closed. Lights off. No bedraggled patients and their caretakers slumping in the waiting room. No fusty odor of despair laced with hope.

"What the hell?" I say and walk toward the front desk. I throw up my hands. "No one bothered to tell me the clinic would be closed today." I peer through the glass in the entry door, hoping to conjure up someone in scrubs. Nada.

"Now what?" says Landon, holding onto Steve's wheelchair. Steve is unusually quiet, has a glazed look in his eyes. Rough night. Landon had to roll out and guide him to the bathroom about once every hour. Lasix works as designed, but cares not a whit for your schedule. Its only purpose in life is to flush out the unwanted fluids. At that, it gets an A+.

Neither Steve nor Landon is fully rested. We need to somehow take care of his lab work and then go home so these boys can sleep. As much as I want to leave, we don't dare move without having his blood drawn.

"Sorry, Sweetie," I say to Steve and pat his arm, "but there's been a glitch. I assumed we were supposed to bring you here as usual, but they appear to be closed. This is Good Friday."

He nods. "Oh."

"Uh, let me think. You gotta have your blood drawn today, that's all there is to it. Ah! Let me call Nelly, your transplant coordinator. She told me she was the one to call if we had a problem. Well, we now have a problem."

I dig through my bag for my cell phone, dial her number and leave a message, saying, "We're here for Steve's blood draw, but you guys are closed. Now what?"

I look at Landon, then at Steve. "Let's go to the ER. They're always open and they can draw his blood there, unless I hear otherwise from Nelly. I don't know why she didn't tell me."

We head off in the direction of the ER, winding through several cold, lonely tiled hallways to get to the other side of the hospital, passing a few people whose leather-soled shoes echo a cavernous click click as they rush by. When we arrive at the ER, Landon locates Steve near a line of empty chairs and sets the brakes. The waiting room is less than a quarter full so far.

Everyone must be in church.

***

I think back to the Middle Eastern, so-called spiritual pilgrimage I signed up for at my then-boyfriend's urging which landed us in the Garden of Gethsemane. Keshavadas was the boyfriend's guru, not mine. And when I scheduled a private consultation before the trip with the guru about whether or not I should go, I started crying at the state of my relationship with the boyfriend. In response, Keshavadas, sitting red-robed and cross-legged on a raised platform in front of me, reached for my hand and placed it over his robes under which his erect penis was raring to go.

This was not the answer I was seeking. I dashed out the door, crying, past his white-robed wife as the guru called out in his gravelly voice, "Come back, my child, come back."

The child did not come back but did go on the trip, having always wanted to see the Pyramids. Dumped the boyfriend later.

Landon talks with Steve while I bring Steve's identification cards to the young man at the Admissions counter to explain the problem—that Steve is a recent liver transplant patient and needs to have his blood checked today, but that the clinic was closed and no one told us. Could they just draw his blood here?

While I'm standing at the counter, I hear Steve saying, "I wanna go home, I wanna go home. Get me a Glucerna." His tone and press of speech worry me. I look over at Landon, puzzled. Landon shakes his head and shrugs his shoulders as if to say, *what's all this?* I gather up the paperwork, stuff it in my bag and sit down next to Steve.

I'm nearly undone by the memories of our last trip to this ER during the evaluation week when the surgical resident would have given Steve heparin if it hadn't intervened.

I'm lucky Steve didn't die on that trip.

I think about the 371,000 people that Johns Hopkins and Harvard Universities say die every year in the United States of "preventable medical errors." If so, that means there are as many as 371,000 friends and/or relatives who grieve every year, unnecessarily.

How many of them are ever told the truth about how their loved one really died?

How do I know this trip to the ER will turn out any better for Steve? We're on the home stretch, literally, hoping to return to California in two or three weeks.

Dammit, I just can't take any more screw-ups.

"I'm sorry, Honey," I say and reach for Steve's shoulder. "We can't go to the apartment just yet. I'm so sorry about that. And I didn't bring a Glucerna. I didn't think we'd be gone this long. But I'm sure they will get to you quickly, and then we can go home and you can have your Glucerna. How's that?"

"I wanna go home now," he says and fidgets in his chair, his pupils dilated and wild.

Landon and I exchange looks.

He moves closer to Steve and says, "It's OK, Dad. This shouldn't take too long, but we've gotta get your blood done today, OK?" I give Landon a thumbs up. He's very kind, like his father, but with more patience.

After thirty minutes of sweet-talking Steve to distract him—"Why don't you tell Landon about Fluffy?"—I return to the Admissions desk. "Excuse me, but Steve needs to have his blood drawn *now*. He's not doing so well; can we please get this done so we can take him home?" The waiting room is now about half full.

The clerk says, "I'll see what I can do." He pages a nurse. She quickly arrives, a small, young woman with a slight limp and a pleasant demeanor. After the clerk has spoken to her, she walks over to us.

"Hi, I'm Ann. So sorry for your wait. I'm going to find you a room so you'll be more comfortable. I'll be right back." She rushes into the bowels of the ER and returns with a smile.

"Follow me," she says and starts off. We follow closely, if slowly.

We arrive at a cold sterile room and I make introductions—Steve, Rosie, Landon.

"Nice to meet you all. Is there anything I can get you, Mr. West, or you, Rosie or Landon?" she says with an endearing smile. Maybe this won't be a disaster after all.

"Steve keeps asking for Glucern," I say. We didn't bring any with us. The only reason we're here is that the Transplant Clinic is closed and no one was there to draw his blood. That's all we need, really, but could you get him a couple of bottles while we're waiting? He's getting more and more agitated, which is not like him. And maybe a couple of blankets? It's pretty cold in here right now."

"Sure. I'll see what I can do," she says. The door hisses shut behind her.

"I wanna lie down," Steve says. He's staring at the exam table. I turn to Landon. "Well, we could do that, yeah? Transfer him to the table so he's more comfortable? I know he still has a sore on his butt. He shouldn't be sitting so much. No telling how long we'll be here."

"Sure," Landon says. He moves Steve's wheelchair closer to the table and sets the brake.

He stands in front of Steve and says, "OK, Dad. I'm gonna help you onto the table. Can you stand up?"

Steve struggles. I know he's trying his best. Landon rushes in to help. "OK, now, Dad. When I count to three, I need you to push." Steve wobbles up on the count of two, but Landon stands prepared and hoists him up and onto the bed.

"Good job, Dad. Now, let's get you to lie down." Landon's kindness brings me to tears.

What would I do without him here?

Steve grumbles but allows Landon to help him get situated. I reach for a pillow lying on top of a nearby cart and hand it to Landon.

"Here you go, Dad, here's a nice pillow. Let's just get your head up a bit so you'll be more comfortable." He slides the pillow in behind Steve's head.

Ann returns with three blankets. "I hope this helps," she says and takes off again. Landon covers Steve with one of them. He knows that Steve often runs hot and might soon kick it off.

Steve mumbles something that resembles, "Thanks," and begins to snore.

"Well, it's good he's so tired. This might be a long wait," I say, sitting next to Landon on a very uncomfortable chair, and wrap the other two blankets around me.

Ann returns with two Glucernas. I thank her.

She says, "There might be a problem with doing a blood draw here. It's only supposed to be done in the Transplant Clinic for transplant patients. I'm going to see if I can reach someone to give me the OK. Sorry about the wait."

"What?" I say. "Blood is blood, right?" I stand up and fidget the kinks out of my back.

"Well, yes, but the transplant department has its own laboratory with special procedures. I need to get permission," she says and scoots out the door.

We're so close to getting out of here. Oh, please God, Angels, Universe, anyone, please help us. I'm a cranky desperado now. I check every hour or so to see what's holding us up.

Finally, four hours later, a technician comes in, draws several vials of Steve's blood. We are soon released to return to the apartment.

I don't remember Eric, the pharmacist, saying anything about the possibility of an allergic reaction to any of the meds Steve is taking.

The Apartment
4:00 p.m.

A new Home Care nurse named Jackie arrives—short, brunette, sunburned.

"Boy, are we happy to see you," I say and tell her what happened last night and in the morning, how Steve seems to have lost some of his mojo, and is having more problems communicating.

"Yeah," says Landon, sitting on the edge of the sofa bed. "He was terribly confused all night when I had to take him to the bathroom about every hour. He didn't seem to know where he was or what was going on."

Jackie nods and walks over to Steve who is sitting in the La-Z-Boy. I introduce Jackie to him.

"How are you doing, Mr. West?" she says, smiling.

"I'm fine. Better wanna go home." I know it is Steve talking, but his spirit has somehow made a getaway. I head toward the bedroom, close the door and sob. We've been so hopeful.

What if the real Steve never returns, but stays in this tangled loop? What if he can never teach again? I have to stop with the scary stories before I wind up in a hysterical puddle. I dry my eyes, wipe my cheeks and return to the living room.

"No place like home, right?" she says to Steve.

"Billy."

Jackie glances at me, nods. She's seen it all before, doesn't judge.

I clear my throat. "Billy is one of our cats who is very attached to Steve. Isn't he, Honey?" I sit on the edge of the sofa bed.

"Billy sleeps with me," Steve says with no affect.

"I know what you mean," says Jackie. "I have three cats. I can't imagine being without them. I did notice a pretty kitty just outside as I walked up. She looked very friendly."

"We call her Fluffy. We'd love to bring her inside, but we can't take a chance on fleas, you know? I do feed her, though. Just can't not help a kitty in need."

"I hear that," she says, turning toward me. Now back to Steve.

"So, Mr. West. I need to take your temperature. Is that OK?" She pulls out the thermometer from her bag.

"Sure." He's smiling, though seemingly unsure about what there is to smile about.

She hands it to Steve. He holds it in his lap, staring at her.

"Hey, Dad," says Landon, "do you need help with that? You know—just open your mouth and put the thermometer in. I know you can do it."

Steve nods and places it in his mouth.

Jackie removes it after a few minutes. "Normal," she says and tucks it into its container.

"Next, I want to check your blood pressure. Can you roll up your shirt sleeve for me?"

"Here, Honey, let me help," I scoot off the bed. I lift his arm and start pushing up his sleeve. Jackie slips the blood pressure cuff on and quickly pumps it up, waits and says, "It's a little high. I'll check with your doctor to see if he wants to increase your blood pressure meds.

"OK, next I need to check your incision to make sure it's not infected or anything. Can you lift up your shirt for me?" Steve is wearing the XXL windowpane, long-sleeved shirt I bought him to accommodate his formerly huge belly. He's now a skinny kid floundering in his father's dress shirt. I need to buy him some clothes to fit his current anorexic frame.

He stares as I lift up his shirt.

Jackie examines it closely. "Looks good!" she pronounces.

"OK, we're almost done. I know this is tiring. I just have a few questions," she says, with all the patience in the world. Nurses should be given the Nobel prize for healthcare.

"Do you know what day it is?"

Steve pauses, looking toward Landon and says, "Sunday."

"OK. Who's the president of our country?"

"Ummm, Bush?"

"OK. Now, let's see if you can get out of the chair by yourself?" Landon moves closer and stands by.

"Yes," he says. He scoots forward and pushes up, almost topples, but Landon catches him.

"That La-Z-Boy is not the easiest thing to get out of, is it?"

"No, it's not. I need a new chair," he smiles.

"Landon, would you please bring over his walker? I want to see how he's doing with it."

Landon moves it in front of Steve who wavers as he stands up to grip it.

"Can you walk down that hallway by yourself?"

Concerned, Landon, moves in to help him.

"That's OK. You can stand near him, but I need to see how much he can do by himself."

Steve sets off, takes a step, stops, another step, stops and so on down the hall. Landon helps him turn around. The same pattern on return.

"OK. Good. That's all today, Mr. West," she says and stands up. "Mary Jane, the nurse who saw you on Wednesday will be back on Monday to check up on you. In the meantime, I want you to continue walking and practicing all of your exercises. Can you do that?"

"Sure."

She walks over to gather her notebooks from the dining room table. She flips through them, turns to me and says, "I can tell from Mary Jane's notes that he's not quite the same now as when she first saw him. That's not uncommon for transplant patients, to lose ground sometimes. They can have ups and downs. Those usually resolve over time. Mary Jane will be coming back to see him on Monday; so that's good. She was just here and saw him when he was feeling better, so she will have something to compare."

I'm tearing up now and say, "Thanks so much for coming today. We really appreciate it." I open the door for her.

"Yes," says Landon, "thank you for coming, Jackie."

Steve waves, "Bye Bye."

So many questions, so few answers, so much worry.

Chapter Fifteen

NOT AGAIN

Saturday, April 4, 2015

I awaken at 12:30 a.m. to a knock on my door. I roll over.
Maybe I'm dreaming. Maybe I can go back to sleep. But, no.
Another knock. Now what? I reach for my glasses, struggle out
of bed, wiggle into my sweatshirt, pants, fleece jacket and open
the door, my heart pounding, my hands clammy. Am I even
breathing?

"What's going on?" I say, opening the door, not wanting to
know. I'm not rested enough for another go-round with liver
catastrophe.

Landon, pacing in the hallway, says, "We've had a terrible
time. He's been babbling all night, not making sense, irritated
about something, don't know what. I could hardly get him to
walk down the hall to the bathroom. He can't seem to keep his
eyes open. I think he hears me but he's not processing well."
Landon wears the frantic look of a mama bear in search of her
cubs.

I pause while I summon my inner caretaker. "I'm so sorry,
Landon. I don't know what to say. This scares the hell out of me."

I pivot toward the living room.

"Nobody said anything about this sort of thing, dammit."

"I'm right with you," he says and follows me down the hall. "Though Jackie did say it happens sometimes that transplant patients have setbacks, remember?"

"I remember. But this doesn't seem like a setback to me. This seems more like Armageddon." I hesitate.

I can't make this all go away when I don't know what the hell is happening. I managed to survive the evaluation week, but in comparison that was kindergarten. This is post-grad territory without the textbooks or the professors.

Who can I turn to?

Steve's confusion, along with his receptive and expressive verbal skills, have worsened by the hour, beginning in the middle of the night last night and continuing all day. And now this.

What the hell?

Earlier in the day, after Jackie left, we had tried to get Steve to eat something, anything—yogurt, Glucerna, hard-boiled eggs. We spent 45 minutes just to make sure he ingested all his evening pills, one swallow at a time. We had to check and re-check to make sure he actually swallowed them.

"Can you open your mouth, Steve? Please open your mouth?" Our cat Billy is notorious for seeming to accept his prednisolone tablet, but spitting it out later. Steve couldn't open his eyes or his mouth without repeated prompting and even then, only for a few seconds.

The pharmacist's words echo again. "There can be no mistakes with his medications."

The surgery to install a new liver was only part of the solution for his presenting health problems. The anti-rejection drugs disarm his body's natural defenses just enough to keep them from destroying his new liver. Without them, all would be lost.

I had to keep telling him, "Steve, Honey, I know you're not feeling well, but you need these pills—you know, the ones that keep your body from rejecting your liver?" He nodded through a brief rent in his fog. My heart breaks to see him like this and to not know if my brilliant, handsome Steve will ever return from wherever the hellhound has kidnapped him.

Steve is behaving more and more as if he's had a stroke or a head injury or a psychotic episode, any one of which would be horrifying. Not to put too fine a point on it, but his symptoms seem to have reached their apotheosis this evening, while we, on the other hand, are sinking to our nadir.

How am I to know that I have not yet reached the outer limits of what Landon and I will be forced to endure?

"This is ridiculous," I say to Landon. "We've got to get him help from someone, somewhere. This can't go on!"

I dash off to my bedroom, grab my phone from the nightstand and dial Nelly's number. Once again, she doesn't answer. Once again, I leave a desperate message. Through my tears, I string together enough words to get her attention, I hope, by ending with, "We're taking him to the emergency room. Please tell one of the transplant surgeons this is all going to hell."

***

It's a painful reminder of the evaluation week when I left messages with the hospital operator, telling her that Steve was in serious cognitive trouble and that he might need Lactulose, and that it was urgent that someone call me back.

Despite the recorded message telling all callers that, "Your call is being recorded for quality assurance purposes," my calls had mysteriously disappeared and the blame shifted to me for supposedly not using the word, "urgent." If only I had used the magic word, they claimed, someone would have burned up the phone lines to reach me Right.

★★★

It occurs to me that the new notebook I had been given might contain some useful information. I discover a phone number for the on call transplant coordinator, whoever she or he may be. I haven't been able to figure out their labyrinthine system of coordinators. It seems that whenever I need them, they are everywhere and nowhere at the same time.

I reach a nurse named Brenda and, after explaining everything in detail, she says, "You need to take him to the ER. I'll alert the transplant team."

Finally!

Saturday, April 4, 2015
2:45 a.m.

After burning up thirty minutes to get Steve dressed—underwear changed ("No, Dad, that foot doesn't go there, it goes here"); pressure socks applied ("Honey, you have to stiffen your leg so we can pull up your socks."); sweat pants pulled on; shirt donned and buttoned; shoes slipped into; laces tied; jacket held open; arms finally slipped inside.

Walking him with his walker to the parking lot; Landon assisting him into the passenger seat of our Kia Rio; Landon folding up the walker and placing it into the trunk. Folding myself, my tote and my worried heart into the back seat.

We're off to a place we know too well. Maybe this time we will get Steve the help he needs? Maybe? I must choose hope, but prepare myself to kick butt if I do not get answers. I know already that I'm going to pay for all this stress after we return to California. I've seen too many caretakers fold from attending to their loved ones as they went through medical hell.

I check us in at the hospital while Landon rolls Steve to the far side of the waiting room. I inform the clerk how seriously ill Steve is, a fresh transplant patient, and that the transplant surgeons would want their patient to be seen right away. The transplant coordinator told me she'd alert the transplant team. I stuff the paperwork into my bag, add it to my growing collection.

"Sure," she says. "I'll try to get someone to see him right away, don't worry." She turns to pick up the phone.

Within thirty minutes, we're called to bring Steve into the patient area of the ER to get set up in a room. A slim, smiling nurse named Wendy comes in and helps Steve out of his clothes and into a gown. She hooks Steve up with an IV, takes his temperature and blood pressure. She asks Steve what's wrong. Silence. Landon and I stand off to the side, watching.

Please Angels, find us someone who can tell us what's going on.

I remove his clothes from the bed and hang them up. I carry his wallet in my fanny pack at all times. He has no need of it right now. Wendy leaves for a minute and brings back a pile of warmed blankets.

"Oh, lucky you, Honey," I say. "Too bad Billy isn't here. He'd love to cuddle with you under those hot blankets, wouldn't he?" Steve smiles and nods.

"Mr. West," Wendy says, "do you know where you are right now?" She's done this countless times with other patients, just a routine night for her. Patience must be her middle name.

"Glucerna," he says and stares at her with his empty eyes, his arms stiff at his sides.

"Can you tell me how you're feeling right now?" Patience again. She's seen it all, heard it twice over.

"I have to pee," Steve says and tears at his gown.

She snatches a urinal off the counter and nods for us to leave while she pulls the curtain around his bed and says, "Here, Mr. West, let me help you."

"Thanks," he says. Even now in the oily gray fog of confusion, my Steve still defaults to politeness. Ever the Midwesterner.

When they're finished, she slides open the curtain again, the high-pitched shrieking of metal against metal. Looks upon us with kindness, probably not thinking what I might be thinking in her place: *poor sucker doesn't know his ass from a teakettle.*

I thank her and introduce Landon.

Just in case she hasn't had a chance to read his medical record, I say, "Steve had a liver transplant on March 17 and did well on the transplant unit. He was discharged just this Wednesday and was doing fine, until Friday when he gradually regressed until now he's almost catatonic. He has trouble opening his eyes and his mouth. Talks in gibberish. We've been having to urge him to drop his jaw just enough to swallow his pills, drink some Glucerna and maybe take a spoonful of yogurt. I brought a list of his medications, in case you need that."

I told myself I wouldn't cry, but I can't help it when I see him lying on the exam table, not knowing how much he's taking in of what I'm saying. I sigh. This is not right, me listing his problems, talking about him in the third person. I would kill to have my first person Steve back again.

Landon, looking lively in spite of his lack of sleep, adds, "I have to take him to the bathroom every hour or so, and when I walk him with his walker down the hall to the bathroom he moves like a snail, can't open his eyes, and I'm not sure he knows what's going on. I have to talk to him constantly to get him to move. He wasn't that way when I first got here on Wednesday night. He looked like hell then because of what he'd been through, but he was talking just fine and making good sense and eating pretty well."

"Thanks for the information," she says and nods. "I will tell the doctor. It will also be in Mr. West's chart."

I also tell her that I made a video of Steve walking down the hallway with Landon and would be happy to share it if that would help them make a diagnosis.

The nurse makes notes as we speak. "OK," she says in a calm way, "I'm going to go get the doctor. It might be a few minutes because we've gotten really busy today." She steps out and hurries down the hall.

Landon and I look at each other, then at Steve who is observing us.

"Dad, Dad, do you know where you are?"

He shakes his head.

"You're in the emergency room at the hospital where you had your transplant," I say. "Remember your liver transplant?"

He nods and pats his belly.

I stand by the bed, massaging his arm. "Your transplant went well, Honey, and you came home to the apartment. Remember? Where Fluffy lives? You were doing great for a while, but then you got sick, so we brought you here because we were so worried."

"I'm fine."

"Well, that's what we're hoping for, that you will be fine again. We're just waiting for the doctor," I say and kiss his cheek.

He smiles and drifts off.

Landon and I step out of the room. He says, "What do you think's going on here?"

"I have no idea. There is such a thing as hospital psychosis, but he was fine when he came home. The only thing that's changed from Thursday to Friday is that Nelly told me to double his Prograf; so," I shrug, "no idea. I'm hoping the doctor can tell us. At this rate, we won't be able to go home to California for who knows how long."

"And I'm scheduled to fly out on Tuesday. I hope he's all better by then," says Landon.

"Oh, I so appreciate your coming, Landon," I say and give him a hug. "I don't know what I would have done without your help. I can't manage him. I talked to the doctors when he was still on the transplant unit about sending him to an in-patient rehab facility for a few days before he came home so he could get stronger and more independent, and they wouldn't do that, I think, because on the unit, he was walking pretty well and making sense. If you hadn't been here now, I would have had to call an ambulance. Like Dan said—he's our local transplant coordinator—the surgeons here are great, but the coordination sucks. Some of Dan's other patients have had similar problems, too, though he didn't provide details. I just don't get it. There's no excuse for this level of disorganization."

I glance down the hall. A tall, stocky man in a white coat is heading our way.

"Hi," he says. "I'm Dr. Thomas." About fifty, some graying at the temples, but with noticeable muscles bulging under his white coat. Maybe he could use the next larger size.

"Hi, I'm Rosie, and this is Steve's son, Landon." He shakes our hands.

"Nice to meet you. Let's go in and I'll take a look at him." We return to Steve's room where he is dozing. I move to his side and shake his shoulder ever so lightly.

"Hey, Steve," I say, "this is Dr. Thomas. He's here to help us figure out what's going on with you."

Steve wakes up and seems more "there." His eyes are brighter and more focused. Maybe the IV has helped. I need to make sure we give him more fluids at home, even if it takes all day.

"Hi," Steve says and smiles. Raises his hand in a slight wave.

"Tell me what's going on, Mr. West," says Dr. Thomas, who is also kind like Wendy. That's a start.

Steve looks at me and then Landon and says, "Well, I've been having trouble with some things."

"Such as?"

"I had a liver transplant."

"Yes, I see that. Do you mind if I look at your abdomen?"

"That's fine."

Dr. Thomas carefully lifts up Steve's gown and looks closely at the incision. Using his stethoscope, he listens as he taps Steve's belly, moves it up to listen to his heart. He slides Steve's gown back down and removes the stethoscope from his ears.

"I'd like to do a CAT scan," he says. "Just to see if there's anything going on that would account for all his symptoms."

"Just so you know, doctor," I say, "we told Wendy that Steve was much better when he came home on Wednesday, seemed like he was on the right track. But, then his Prograf was doubled late Thursday afternoon. Would that have anything to do with this?"

I watch him carefully for any signs of recognition. None.

"I'm not sure," he says. "Clearly something's not right. I'm going to go order the CAT scan now. They might be awhile since we're pretty busy, but I will get the results tonight and let you know. The nurse will be back in to see if you need anything." He steps out into the hallway.

"Oh, one more thing," I say. "Before his transplant, at home, Steve had difficulty with hepatic encephalopathy. We used Lactulose at first, but then switched to Xifaxan and were told not to use both at the same time. But when we were here for the evaluation week, we had forgotten his Lactulose, and he became very disoriented. Not as bad as he is now, at least then he could walk and talk past his confusion. I don't know if that helps at all."

"We'll wait to see what the CAT scan tells," Dr. Thomas says and smiles. "I'll come back when the results are in. Take care." I watch him stride down the hallway. He talks good, he looks good.

"Well, he was nice, right?" I say. Landon nods, crossing his arms over his chest, nodding his head in a hopeful manner.

"Did you bring any Glucerna?" Steve says.

"Yes, I did, but I'll have to make sure it's OK for you to have it now. You're getting a CAT scan, and I think they don't want you to have anything besides water. Sorry."

He frowns. "When's the CAT scan?"

"I'm not sure, Honey, it might be a while. They seem pretty busy."

Wendy returns to ask if we need anything. I tell her about Steve and Glucerna.

She shakes her head. "No, sorry, he can't have it right now, but he can have small sips of water."

Two hours later, the attendant enters, says his name is Bruce and that he's here to wheel Steve down to Radiology. We step aside, let him release the brakes and Steve's IV. I move toward him, planning to accompany Steve to the exam.

Bruce says, "You guys should stay here, it's pretty tight quarters in the scan room. We'll take good care of him."

I lean in and give Steve a kiss. "OK, Honey, you're going to get your CAT scan now and as soon as the doctor gives us the results, we can go home to the apartment."

"Right-o," he says, giving me a thumbs up. At last, a spark of humor.

I watch Bruce carefully wheel Steve down the hallway. My stomach churns whenever Steve is out of my sight. I chew on my lip and do some shoulder rolls.

Landon and I head to the cafeteria for a quick snack; we talk about nothing in particular. It's tough living in the All-Steve-All-the-Time show.

When we return, Bruce is wheeling Steve back to his room.

Two hours later, Dr. Thomas returns.

"Nothing out of line on Mr. West's CAT scan," he tells us. "You can take him home."

"But, but, don't you want to keep him in the hospital to run some more tests?" I say tamping down my querulousness. "He's perked up a bit since we got here. Maybe the IV fluids helped, but still, he's not the same as he was on Wednesday when he first came home."

"No, I don't think it's necessary for him to stay in the hospital," he says and leaves.

Easy for him to say; he doesn't have to live with him.

I could kick myself for not urging him to watch the videos. I should have been more aggressive, but in the medical world, there's a fine line—when and how much to push; when to be quiet.

I might have chosen the wrong option.

Landon turns to me and says, "What are we going to do if Dad doesn't get any better than this?"

Tears shimmer as I say, "I can't take care of him at home in the state he's in right now. He'd have to go to a nursing home. But since we're not rich, he'd soon end up needing a Medicaid bed, and those facilities are rank beyond belief and not some place you'd ever want to send a loved one."

He crosses his arms over his chest, his face etched with sadness.

"Look, Landon, I know you're supposed to leave on Tuesday, but I'd really like you to reschedule that. I can't deal with him alone, not when he's like this, and I don't know when or if he will get better."

"Uh," he says, pauses and looks at the floor. "I don't know."

"Please, Landon, please. I can't handle your Dad by myself!"

"I'll call my boss tomorrow."

"All right. Thanks!"

What will I do if Landon can't stay? I do not want to think about that right now.

***

Many years ago, I received a rare letter from my father. I had just finished my degree in psychology and my then-husband Don had the summer off from his college teaching job. Don answered an ad in the *New York Times* for a young couple to spend the summer on Long Island with a wealthy family, helping out with cooking and working on the grounds.

We got the job, being the hearty, honest Midwesterners this old-money New York couple had grown fond of from previous summer hires. We drove from Illinois to Sands Point, Long Island, where they paid us well for the summer.

I wrote home once that I was exhausted from having to cook all day. My eighth-grade drop-out father actually wrote back and shocked me by saying of my exhaustion, that "God broadens the back to bear the burden."

This was rich coming from the man who never went to church or, as far as I knew, never believed in God.

I wanted to, but didn't, write back to say "Why doesn't God just relieve you of the damn burden?"

Chapter Sixteen

WHAT FRESH HELL IS THIS?

Saturday, April 4, 2015
7:00 a.m.

W e stumble into the apartment, our spirits flagging from our latest hospital adventure, hoping for nothing more than a good long nap. Even though Landon is young, the nascent bags under his eyes bespeak the toll his dad's illness is exacting. It must be painful for him to see his dad debilitated, although he doesn't say.

Steve has always been strong, fit, loquacious—the one who taught Landon how to ski, how to drive a stick shift, and who modeled kindness. Now Steve is skinnier than a mannequin and not able to help even himself.

"We're home, Honey," I say to Steve. "Did you notice Fluffy waiting for you? I'm going to give her some food in a minute. Maybe later we can go out and pet her a bit. She seems to enjoy that a lot. Want to?"

Landon stands by as Steve shuffles with his walker toward the sofa bed.

"Do you want to lie down?" Landon asks his Dad.

"Yes." I help Landon remove Steve's jacket and shoes and set them under the desk.

"Are you hungry, Darlin'?" I sigh, knowing that this is going to be another damn struggle. We're just not able to get enough real food into him to stem the weight loss. I have stocked the refrigerator with his favorites, but never mind. I told Landon to make sure he helps himself to whatever he finds, just stay away from my mint chip ice cream. There's plenty of vanilla and chocolate.

Steve nods and turns over to hug the stuffed, fuzzy beige bunny Landon and his kids gifted him for Easter.

"I'll go get him some yogurt. He needs to have something more than the Glucerna," Landon says and heads for the kitchen.

"Thanks, Dude."

Landon returns with a bowl and plops down next to Steve, who is now sitting upright on the edge of the bed, feet on the floor.

"Hey, Dad, want some yogurt?" He holds out a spoonful.

"Yogurt." He turns his head toward Landon.

"Can you open your mouth?" Landon raises the spoon and waits for Steve to respond.

Steve nods, his eyes closed, but doesn't open his mouth.

"Can you open your mouth, Sweet Pea?" I say, from the kitchen. Landon's got some good yogurt for you."

I'm recording a video of this interaction. I'm determined to find some way to convey Steve's problems to his doctors. I hope that seeing the videos will trigger an "A-ha" moment and that the doctor will hit his forehead with the heel of his hand and cry, "Oh, of course. Why didn't we think of that sooner?"

This can't go on.

Slowly, Steve's mouth opens a crack. Landon slides the spoon in. "Good. Now, can you swallow it?"

Landon turns and says to me, "Even when he gets it into his mouth, it's like he can't swallow, or he can't do it unless I ask him."

Steve finally swallows.

"Good job, Dad. How about another bite?"

Landon repeats and repeats and repeats until Steve has finally eaten half a container.

I turn off the video recorder.

The two of us spend another forty-five minutes encouraging him to swallow his pills. Whatever it takes.

"Good job, Steve, you did it!" I say and give him a kiss.

Steve cuddles up with the little stuffed bunny hugging his face. Landon sits back down at the foot of the bed.

I turn the video recorder back on.

(Note to reader: What follows are Steve's exact words, transcribed from the video.)

Steve rolls over, puts pillows under his head and says to Landon, "Push it up toward you and we're gonna make a, we're gonna make a pillow, a new pillow and now and now Landon and segment and pillow."

Landon glances over at me. I shake my head. "This is called 'word salad.' It can happen in schizophrenia, head injury or stroke or some other kind of neurological problem. The CAT scan didn't show a stroke or head injury. That leaves maybe some kind of psychosis? Damned if I know."

Steve continues, staring at Landon and waving his hands in the air. "OK. We're going to put three of these together so we have a segment, OK, follow me? No, sorry, Landon, which is you, OK?"

"OK." Landon's playing along.

Steve looks over at me and continues with his pantomime. "I'm gonna make this long what I'm doing is making it long, so it will be open and I can swallow and talk, see what I mean?" Steve's earnestness in making his presentation saddens me.

The poor guy doesn't know what the hell he's talking about.

Landon: "Uh-huh."

"Stay with me now," Steve continues. "I'm combining Landon, segment and pillow into one pillow and I'm going to put a solid iron bar on the right side of this pillow, OK? Third bar, going to pull that through, OK?" He gestures with his hands, certain of the reality of what he's describing.

"I'm pulling it through, OK? Now we got a new pillow. Now I'm going to chew a new pillow; actually all I have to do is chew it hard so, but it's open."

"OK, Dad. Sounds like you're all set." Landon wants to support his Dad, but it ain't easy.

"All set," Steve says and scoots down under the covers with his bunny, rolls over and begins to snore. I turn off the recording.

"I'm going to show this performance to his doctors, and if that doesn't give them a clue about his problems, I don't know what will," I say. "I don't know about you, but I need a long, long nap. Do you think you can sleep, Landon? We've been up for way too long."

"Good idea," Landon says and smooths out the sheets on his bed.

I head off to my bedroom. Don't want to call or email anyone. What could I say: "Steve is crazy and no one seems to know what's wrong or care enough to find out?" I'm still hopeful, don't know why. Probably because the alternative is unthinkable. I crack open the novel, *Woman on the Train,* which I checked out from the local library during a rare free moment. The staff had no problem giving me, an out-of-stater, a library card.

Librarians and nurses should rule the world.

I've loved libraries and librarians ever since I was a kid. Our small town library was only a few skips away. A place of magic. They actually gave you books to take home! And when you returned them, they gave you more. For free!

★★★

Several years ago I wrote and recorded a short piece about my love of libraries for the San Francisco NPR affiliate, KQED-FM, in their Perspective Series. "Safe Haven" won the Listener Favorite Award, but better than that, I heard from several librarians about how much they loved the piece:

"Two weeks ago I went to the Berkeley Public Library to get a new library card. After completing the application I headed for the 'Help Desk.' The young man seated behind the counter looked no more than twenty, with dreadlocks trailing down to his waist.

As a child, I had never heard of the word, "dreadlocks," but I would have known whom to ask—either Miss Esther or Miss Florence Johnson, spinster sisters who presided over our small Illinois town library with firm and knowing hands.

It was in this building that I learned I could travel anywhere in my mind. As long as I asked with sufficient respect, Esther and Florence were willing to point the way to whatever world called me.

They never knew how much that tall skinny tomboy craved the quiet protection of the library—a respite from her cramped home filled with unacknowledged longings, regrets, and the smoke from her dad's unfiltered Pall Mall cigarettes. And besides, there were RULES. No one could hit me while I was in the library. No one could yell at me or call me "Dunce." For me it was like skidding into home plate with the umpire yelling, 'SAFE!'

I thought back to that time as I walked toward the Help desk with my finished paperwork and was blindsided by a flutter of tears. What would I have become if I hadn't been able to hide out in that library to read, to dream and most of all to be safe? And what about all those young people I saw in the alcoves, sitting quietly with their books? Where would they be if they didn't have their library?

I brushed aside my tears and inhaled deeply while the young man entered my information into his computer. When he looked up and handed me the new card, he flipped his dreadlocks over his shoulder and said, 'Oh, and if you lose it, it'll cost you $1.00 to get a new one.'"

"Don't worry," I said fighting a new wave of tears, "I've never lost one yet."

***

In bed, I begin to read the novel and am thankfully swept away into the troubles of other folks. What's going on here? What's this character thinking? How is she going to get out of this mess?

Anything to take me away from the hospital and release me from this crazy train.

I rise around noon, check in on the boys.

Landon sighs and says, "He's keeping up the word salad or gibberish or whatever you want to call it. And he's been grunting and moaning."

What can you say? You've got nothing for him. The phone rings. You zip to the bedroom to answer.

It's Nelly.

She says, "I got your message. What's going on?"

"Well, first off, we went to the Transplant Clinic to get his blood drawn on Friday, but it was closed for Good Friday. No one told me about that."

"No, it wasn't closed. There was someone there to draw blood."

"What? No lights were on, no people around, I looked in the window but didn't see anyone. Why didn't you tell me?"

"They were in there. All you had to do was knock."

"Now how would I have known that?"

"I don't know, but they were there."

"Are you aware that we ended up in the ER for several hours because no one bothered to tell me that? They weren't even going to draw his blood in the ER, but they must have gotten hold of someone in your department, because they finally did the draw. This was very hard on Steve to end up in the ER for so many hours. Inexcusable."

"Well, they were there." Silly me; hell would freeze over before I heard so much as *I'm so sorry* from that woman.

"OK," I say, "so what about tomorrow? Easter Sunday. Is someone going to be there at 8:30 in the morning?" I shift from one foot to the other. It's exhausting to keep my inner sailor from firing off a string of expletives. I know it's kind of cheesy, but Steve and I love to swear when we're home alone. He comes from a Brethren background with a strict dad who believed swearing was the work of the devil. I went to Lutheran Sunday school, Bible school in the summers and church on Sundays. I liked the music and the Golden Rule, but the rest? Not so much.

"Of course. Just knock on the door," Nelly says without a dollop of kindliness.

"By the way," I continue, "did you get the message that we had to take Steve to the ER again yesterday? Our second trip in less than two days? He's behaving kind of crazy, not making any sense. Did you see the note that he had a CAT scan? Can you please talk to his surgeons about this?"

I pause, take a deep breath and stress, "*Something is wrong.* Steve was fine when he came home from the hospital, but then you upped his Prograf. Could that have anything to do with Steve's crazy behavior?"

"I'll talk with his doctor." She says and hangs up. I stand still with my phone in my raised hand.

Take one very deep breath, Rosie.

Well, that went well. I swear, if I could have reached through the phone line to wring her neck, I might have done.

If this were fiction, I would have to bestow upon Nelly some redeeming qualities—say, she's a Big Sister for a homeless girl, or say that instead of tossing her yappy, pooping, peeing puppy into the dumpster, she delivers him to a shelter—but this ain't fiction and real people do not always hew to my values of kindness and respect.

Easter Sunday, April 5, 2015
3:00 a.m.

When we were kids, our mother made my brother and me go with her to church every Sunday, whether we liked it or not. As a teen, I didn't mind going to communion because the minister's older son, David, upon whom I had a gigantic crush, helped his father serve the tiny glasses of Mogen David—a communion barista, if you will—to the kneeling parishioners. I loved the sickly sweet burn as it oozed all the way down, lighting up my innards like a glow stick.

If Jesus could rise again, maybe there would be hope for Steve. Or not.

I'm awakened at 3:00 a.m. to the sound of—what? Steve grunting? I slip into my robe, rush down the hall.

"He's still crazy," says Landon, sitting on the edge of his bed, disheveled and yawning.

"He's been hollering 'Glucerna, Glucerna, Glucerna,' for about an hour. He's also been moaning."

"Oh, crap. I don't know what more to do," I say to Landon. "I'm sorry you didn't get any sleep."

"Steve, Honey, what's going on?" I say, turning to him.

"Glucerna. Glucerna." He's a 78-rpm record with a needle skip.

"Yes, yes, we hear you, but can you stop hollering? It's 3:00 o'clock in the friggin' morning, Steve. Landon needs his sleep, and you need your sleep."

I suddenly recall that Steve brought his Restoril with him. I paw through his ditty bag, clutch the bottle. Select one pill and sit on the edge of the bed with a bottle of Glucerna in my hand.

"You can have some Glucerna, Steve, if you promise to swallow this pill to help you sleep? Can you do that?" Steve nods.

"Good. Now, I need you to open your eyes, can you open your friggin' eyes, Sweetheart? I know you can do it, please open your eyes." I can tell he's trying, his muscles are twitching, his eyes peeking out from his prison through small slits.

"OK. Great. Now, open your mouth so you can take this pill. I'll give you some Glucerna to wash it all down." Steve doesn't move.

"Landon, can you help?"

Landon comes over and sits next to Steve.

"Come on, Dad. You've got to open your mouth and take this pill so you can get some sleep. Can you do that, Dad? Please?"

I move in carefully and touch Steve on his chin and say, "This is your chin. We need it to slide down so you can take your pill." Movement happens. Yay. I put the pill on his tongue, give him a bottle of Glucerna. "Now tip that up and swallow . . . swallow." He swallows. Touchdown!

"Thank God. We knew you could do it, Sweetie!" I thrust my fist into the air.

***

We are living in liminal limbo—Steve and Landon and I. Will Steve die/will he not? Can Rosie pass under the ever-lowering bar without pitching to the ground?

Reminds me of the time I embarked on a sailing trip at 31 with four other women around the British and American Virgin Islands. The Basa Anderea, a gleaming 63 ft. wooden sailing vessel, built by the Vanderbilt family in the 20s, now a tourist boat, became our water-borne home for two weeks.

Vance and Alice, seasoned skippers and cooks, catered to our whims—"Keep the Piña Coladas coming!"—as we sailed into St. Croix, Little Dix, St. John's, Peter Island, Virgin Gorda, Tortola, and our home port of St. Thomas. Ah, the Sweet Carelessness of Youth. We all took seriously the directive, "Come to de Islands, Mon" and could have compiled a guide book to the best rum, coconut and pineapple drinks in the Caribbean.

On the next to last evening in Charlotte Amalie, capital of St. Thomas, Sheila, Barb and I taxied to Club Zulu which opened onto a narrow cobblestone alley.

Inside, blue smoke wafted from one end to the other of the blackened room, the beat of Bob Marley's sinuous reggae promising an evening of no regrets.

It was nearing midnight. Just as we were downing the last of our libations, vowing to return one day, the music lowered and a man's deep accented voice cut in to announce, "Are you ready for de Limbo Contest? Only pretty woman come to de dance floor." Barb, Sheila and I squirmed and lowered our heads as we cast sneaky glances at each other. *No way.* The spotlight sailed around the room, training on one woman at a time.

"You. You will come to de dance floor."

One by one, four women wobbled to the center of the room, lining up willy nilly behind the newly set up limbo bar, shivering with excitement or was that panic?

Then the spotlight landed on me. Piña-ed by my Coladas, there was no time to wonder was I too drunk or not drunk enough as I shuffled toward the limbo line in my short shorts and my "I Slept on a Virgin" t-shirt.

Was I about to set a new personal best for stupid?

Reggae exploded, with its steady up-stroke of rhythm guitar, aka, the "skank beat." Not that we were skanks. Five women, giggling, joking behind our hands, "What were we thinking?"

Too late to back out now!

We swayed to the music as one brave woman after another set off and cleared the bar. I'd been working out at the gym, so no sweat until the bar was lowered and then lowered again, winnowing the field down to two.

The other woman had boobs with a life of their own—difficult to say how many cups' worth. While she was bending backward, headed under the bar, they remained standing.

And that's how I won a bottle of Scotch on a hot summer's eve in the balmy Caribbean.

***

And that's how it's been with Steve—me bending over backwards as far as I can go to save his life. The only prize I want is for him to live.

I'm not sure how to make that happen. Why aren't they telling me what's wrong? They don't seem impressed or interested even when I explain the weird changes in Steve.

Their lack of curiosity is puzzling. No one has wanted to watch the videos I've recorded—one of which shows him unable to walk with his walker down the hall normally, even with Landon's guidance. He's unable to follow directions, unable even to open his eyes. The other one shows Steve in full word salad mode, the vegetables flying freely.

Wouldn't you think that if they didn't know what was wrong, they'd want to see the videos? Especially if they didn't know what was wrong. They should be eager and grateful, even, to gather more evidence so as to make a diagnosis.

Or do they really know what's going on but for some godforsaken reason, don't want us to know, don't want to tell me?

I've since read that one of the hallmarks of medical gaslighting is withholding information from the patient and/or family.[9,10,11]

If that's what was happening, how could I find out, and moreover what, if anything could I do about it?

How much longer are we going to be forced to put up with this horror show?

Easter Sunday, April 5, 2015
8:30 a.m.

Off to the lab for more blood work. We make it to the Transplant Clinic on time; the waiting room is still empty, no lights. I knock on the door as Nelly suggested. Sure enough, a young man appears at the door, leads us back to the lab and draws several vials of blood. Even though Steve's brain is not firing on all cylinders, he can still cooperate. We return to the apartment and to bed.

Later, we struggle to help him eat. Nothing's improved. Can't open his eyes. Can't open his mouth. He has moved on, though, from "Glucerna" as the focus of his perseveration to "Clausen," as in pickles. I would love to peek into that brain to observe whatever gavotte those synapses are performing.

No matter what it is, it has to stop soon or we will never make it back to California.

Chapter Seventeen

A MIRACLE, ANYONE? ANYONE?

Monday, April 6, 2015

Another day, another Glucerna. When will this end? I'm looking forward to the Home Care nurse's visit today. Mary Jane, the nurse who first evaluated Steve after his discharge from the transplant unit, is arriving at 1:00 p.m. I hope she notices Steve's marked deterioration—how could she not?—and can give us advice about what to do.

I utter a silent prayer: *Please, Angels, we need a miracle. We can't take much more of this.* Silly me. No amount of reading or in-person explanations about the transplant process could have prepared me for this. I hadn't expected such a tsunami. I've been chugging down the ibuprofen, icing my neck, putting heat on my back, trying to keep the old bod together until I can return home. Landon is already up, or rather, he's hardly been to bed since he arrived.

Steve is a 24/7 project. How could I have managed him alone? Even with Landon's help, the exhaustion is profound. Slumped at the desk in my bedroom, my lazy eyes gazing out the open window at the little lizard clinging to the screen, it occurs to me that I could simply cry uncle and leave, just like that. Call Southwest Airlines, make a reservation, pack a small bag, taxi to the airport and be gone.

What are they gonna do? Arrest me? I almost don't care.

But now I hear Steve calling for me and I rush back to the living room.

Landon is once again coaxing Steve to eat, and drink. I head to the counter to prepare Steve's pills, take them to Landon and say in my jokey way, "Let's see how long it takes *this* time."

My humor falls flat, even for me.

We repeat and repeat and repeat, and finally the pills are floating in Steve's innards, ready to do battle. If only there were a pill for my battle.

Mary Jane, the home care nurse, arrives and rings the doorbell. I rush to the door.

"You-have-no-idea-how-glad-we-are-to-see-you."

She registers my near-hysteria and asks, "What's going on?"

"We don't friggin know. We've been to the ER twice, and no one can tell us what might be happening. He talks like a crazy person, can't eat or drink or walk well with his walker. Talks in word salad. He's just not right and, uh," I sniff, "uh, we don't know what to do." I blow my nose and cough.

I stand frozen as she walks over to Steve who is still sitting on the edge of the bed.

"Hello Mr. West, remember me?"

"Glucerna." He says, his eyes dull.

"Yes, Glucerna. You like that, right?

"Glucerna."

"Do you know where you are, Mr. West?" she asks with all the patience in the world.

"Bunny."

I hurry over to the bed and root through his sheets to find his stuffed bunny, and hand it to him.

He grabs it and says, "My bunny," and hugs it to his face.

"Landon brought that for Steve for Easter Sunday," I say.

"It's beautiful," she says. "Do you have a name for him?"

"Bunny."

"Can you get up and walk for me, Mr. West?" She points to his walker. Landon swings it over.

"Landon," Steve says, jerking his pale puny arms and legs, but not getting up.

"Do you want me to try and walk him?" asks Landon.

"Yes, please, if you can." How can she remain so calm?

"OK. Dad. We're gonna take a walk to the bathroom. Can I help you up?"

Steve looks up at Landon, then at the walker and begins to push with his legs. Landon grabs him under his arms and hoists him to standing position behind the walker.

"Good job. Are you ready, Dad? Let's go." Steve stands still, looking around, eyes unfocused.

"Come on Dad, you know how to do this, remember? We do it all the time. Take one step, then another and another? You know, like this." Landon lifts one leg, then another, pantomiming walking.

"That's OK," Mary Jane says. "He can sit back down. I've seen enough."

She walks to her bag and pulls out her cell phone, saying to us,

"This is terrible. When did it start?"

"Uh, well, he got home on Wednesday," I say, "when you first saw him, and he seemed to be doing well. We took him for his blood draw on Thursday morning. Nelly called Thursday afternoon and said to increase the Prograf. He's been sliding downhill ever since."

She nods. "I think you should take him back to the ER. I'm going to call Nelly."

Oh, joy! Another round of who-the-hell-knows what's wrong with Steve? Landon looks alarmed.

Nelly answers. We can only hear Mary Jane's side of the conversation. "Mr. West has deteriorated since I saw him last Wednesday. He can't talk, can barely stand up, and this has been going on for several days. He needs to be seen right away. Something is very wrong." She listens quietly to Nelly's response.

"Uh, yes, that's what I'm recommending, but are you going to have one of his transplant surgeons see him when he arrives? I think they would be appalled to see him now."

Mary Jane shakes her head and frowns. "So, that's it? Just to go to the ER and check in? But are you going to alert the transplant surgeons or not?" Mary Jane's words emerge crisp and contained.

"OK," she says. "I'll tell them that." She hangs up.

Mary Jane turns to us and says, "She wants you to take him to the ER. But, first I want to take his blood pressure, his temperature and examine his abdomen." She does this with Steve's cooperation. While they're occupied, I rush to the bedroom and grab my tote bag, haul it to the kitchen, throw in a Glucerna, some nuts, a sandwich, some crackers, a bottle of green tea. Too bad I can't pack up my mint chip ice cream.

Will this lunacy never end?

Mary Jane finishes, stands up and says, "Well, I'm sorry this has happened. I hope he gets better."

"Thank you *so* much. Um, I couldn't help notice, uh, but it sounded to me like Nelly was sort of rude to you on the phone. She's been nothing but rude to us since we got here."

Her lips twist into a half-smile, she nods and says, "Good luck."

I hug her on her way out the door and say, "Thank you so much." I hang on a bit too long. She's the first one to give voice to our fears.

We corral Steve into his pressure socks, shoes, jacket and scoot him out the door and into the car.

What fresh hell awaits us this time?

***

I wonder why I was so slow to consider that the medical staff might be gaslighting us—deliberately withholding the reason for Steve's crazy behavior. That would explain the dissembling I was dimly aware of every time I asked a direct question. But why? Why would they not want to tell us what was causing Steve's symptoms and then do something about them?

I could kick myself for not catching on sooner. I was trained in psychotherapy, for godsakes. I should have suspected. I'll never forgive myself. I have no defense other than to say Landon and I have both been knackered, frightened, and maybe a bit addled, if you want to know the truth.

But who would ever think that a physician would choose to withhold the truth? It makes no sense, especially since the truth is hurting their patient, not to mention his family.

They are aware of it, yet doing nothing? I've not exactly been subtle about explaining all the weird shit we've faced while trying to take care of Steve. In fact it seems as though they're going out of their way to ignore us; otherwise why are they refusing to acknowledge our distress?

I've got to get to the bottom of this, no matter what. It's crazy that they would allow Steve and Landon and me to suffer.

What long-term damage might haunt Steve for the rest of his life because of their ignorance or dissembling or whatever the hell it is that they are doing?

Chapter Eighteen

Is There No One to Help?

Monday, April 6, 2015
3:00 p.m.

Emergency Room again. We should be getting Frequent Bat-Crap-Crazy-Miles. I hope the third time's the charm, because there's only so much more of this Landon and I can take. But of course, we will "take" whatever we have to in order to wring answers out of someone, anyone, who can help Steve. If his current state does not improve by next Tuesday when Landon returns to Los Angeles, I won't be able to care for him myself.

And then what?

Who at this hospital is going to go to bat for us? I have yet to meet that person. We've been tossed into the deep end of the shark tank while onlookers, clutching lifesaving ring buoys, stand by and stare.

At last, Steve's name is called. Landon pushes him toward the nurse holding the door open. Emma leads us down the hall and around the corner to a private room. Same old, same old. Gown, BP, temp, IV, oxygen, blood draw. "The doctor will be in to see you soon." As usual, bless his heart, Steve cooperates with the poke. I'm surprised he has any veins left.

"Sorry about all of this," I say to Steve and wave my hand around. "We're just doing our best to find out why you're having so many problems." He nods.

Landon brought along Steve's bunny and cuddles it next to Steve's face. Steve's eyes open and a sweet, child-like smile rolls in.

"There you are," I say. "That's my Honey. You got your bunny, Honey. He'll keep you safe and sound. That's what bunnies do, right?" Even to myself I'm sounding unhinged, but I'll do anything to pry him out of his fog.

The nurse returns. "Is there anything I can get you while you wait?"

"I think he might have to pee. He's been squirming around. Sweetie, do you have to pee?"

Steve nods. "Yes."

"He's on Lasix, still, and you know how that goes." I smile and shrug, trying to make light and do a little bonding with the hard-working nurse.

"Sure. Why don't you step outside while I help him?" She closes the door.

"So, what do you think?" says Landon, arms folded across his chest. I know he'd like some hopeful news. We scoot back as other patients are wheeled past us, one looking particularly forlorn.

"Well, we're here again," I say. "I'm going to ask that they contact one of Steve's transplant surgeons to come and see him. Those guys know what he was like before the surgery, so they should have an idea of why he's changed so dramatically."

Landon nods. "Sounds like a plan."

"The only one I've got right now, I'm afraid," I sigh. Sighing is what I do now. A regular old sighing machine.

Emma opens the door. "You can go in now."

"Oh," I say, "before I forget, he's been complaining about the sore on his butt. We didn't think to bring his special cream, could you please get him some? I'm sorry, but I can't remember the name of it."

"I'll check his chart and see what I can do." She smiles as she heads toward the door.

"Thank you so much." Maybe we can relax, now? Maybe we're in good hands?

I turn to Steve, lean in and give him a kiss. "Hey, there, how's it going, Big Guy? You look like you're having too much fun with that bunny." Steve cozies up and nuzzles his little fuzzy companion.

Landon laughs. "Hey, Dad, you'd better watch out for those little brown smarties!"

Steve catches the joke and laughs for the first time in days. It seems that every time he's given IV fluids he perks up. That makes sense. We've not been successful getting him to drink much, let alone eat.

"I asked Emma to get you some of that butt cream they gave you on the transplant unit. I'm sorry I didn't think to bring it with me."

You sigh and shake your head. You've been on red alert for the past four months. You can't think of everything.

Landon, standing near, launches into a nursery rhyme, "Hey, Dad, remember this?" he says, with gusto, "Slug-a-bed, Slug-a-bed barley butt."

Steve rides the wave with Landon, "Your bum is so heavy you can't get up." They laugh. Father and son out for a good time.

"That's hilarious," I say. "You guys should take your show on the road." I'm bouncing on my feet, trying to stay awake.

They repeat and repeat. Whatever works, right?

Emma returns. "I'm sorry, I checked, but we don't have any of that cream here."

"What?" I say and move forward. "This is an emergency room, can't you get some from the pharmacy?"

"I'm sorry, I was told no." She looks genuinely embarrassed to have to tell me that as she leaves.

"Oh, for Pete's sake," I say and snap. "That's ridiculous." I know it's not her fault, but geeze-louise, this is getting old. "What the fuck?" I turn to Landon.

"Steve's in pain and they can't get his fucking butt cream? This is un-fucking-believable."

I laugh when I recall one of Steve's lectures on "infixes." An "infix," in contrast to a prefix or suffix, is a new grammatical feature of English vocabulary. It's a word stuck right in the middle of another word, mostly commonly featuring the word "fuck."

"I know, weird, huh? Oh, wait!" I say. "I know where I can get some. Stay here. I'm gonna run up to the transplant unit. They'll have it." I take off at a run.

My New Balance kicks cradle my feet as I leap two stairs at a time, race down the hall, reach the transplant unit, whirl this way and that to find a nurse. I skid round the corner and there, at an isolated counter sit two nurses doing their charting, one of them Karen, the slim brunette and the best nurse Steve had had while on the unit.

Karen looks up and says, "Hi, Rosie. What are you doing here?"

I stop. So good to see a friendly face. I throw up my hands and say, "Trying to get some of Steve's butt cream. They don't have it in the ER and apparently can't get it, so I thought I'd come up here." Karen is so kind, I can't hold back the tears. She introduces me to blond forty-something Sharon, who works on the unit, too.

Noting my distress, Karen asks, "Why is he in the ER?"

"Well," I snuffle and struggle to hold it together. "This is the third time in three days we've had to take him to the ER. We're trying to figure out what's wrong. He's gone crazy—word salad—can barely open his eyes, has trouble opening his mouth so we can barely feed him, can't walk without help. He wasn't like this when he first came home and then they increased one of his meds; and now, I can't get anyone to tell me what's wrong."

"That's Prograf," say Karen and Sharon in unison. "We see that all the time. We never had a problem with Cyclosporine, which is what they used before Prograf came on the scene."

"What? Why hasn't anyone told us?" I wipe the snot from my nose with the back of my hand.

"Look," Karen says, "I don't know why they didn't tell you it's Prograf—they have their reasons, I guess—but, if I were you, I would ask them to change him to Cyclosporine. But please don't tell them I told you that!"

I'm gobsmacked. My brain chirrs, struggling to rearrange the neurons of understanding. *What did I just hear?* That it's so obvious to them that it's Prograf, and yet they haven't even seen Steve since he was discharged?

So why isn't it obvious to anyone else? Why do the docs not own up to it and change his meds? Why put Steve and us through this hell?

Nothing makes sense, nothing.

"That's right," Sharon says. "Cyclosporine was great, but then, they made a change, who knows why? Guess Prograf was the shiny new thing." She hands me a tube of Steve's butt cream.

"Thanks so much, you guys. You may have just saved Steve's life!" I hug them again.

I rush to retrace my steps back down to the ER, giving a triumphant swing to the tube of butt cream when I tell Landon what I found out about Prograf.

"Oh, Christ. Why didn't anyone tell us that?" Landon says.

"That, my dear Landon, is the $64,000 dollar question." I take a deep breath to calm down. I don't know how much more of this I can endure. Or how much more Steve can take.

Feels as though a Gatling gun has been firing at us, one deadly round after another, for days.

What damage is this drug doing to him?

Steve looks peaceful with his bunny resting next to his cheek, but all of a sudden his legs and arms fall rigid, as if he's had a fright. He starts groaning and shaking all over, with his head rearing back, mouth hanging open, an equal measure of choking and groaning. Now his legs and arms begin jerking.

"Shit! Your Dad's having a seizure!" I scream and skid over to Steve and—I know you're not supposed to do this, but this is not a clinical class, this is my Steve and I need to save him, fuck the class—I stick my hand in his mouth, reach for his tongue so he can breathe.

"Go get help! He's having a seizure!" It lasts barely an agonizing minute, maybe not even that, but I've aged ten years in those scant seconds. Steve is out of it, probably doesn't even know what hit him.

A young male nurse named John strolls in with Landon and says, "No, he's not having a seizure. We have him wired up, and he showed no evidence of seizure activity."

"Well, what do you call it? I've seen seizures and this looked to me like a tonic-clonic seizure, no matter what your machine tells you!" I've lost it now.

He shakes his head and leaves.

Just as I'm about to go to scout out and kidnap one of the transplant surgeons, if it kills me, Steve starts seizing again, only milder this time. I keep my fingers away from his throat and don't even bother screaming for a nurse.

Emma hurries in and quietly adds some sort of sedative to his IV.

"That should help," she says. I don't even ask.

I tell Landon to keep an eye on Steve. "I've got to *do* something, dammit! I will *not* let him die."

Feeling like a kitten tossed into a dryer, tumbling and tumbling and tumbling, screaming for help, *Someone get me outta here!* I shove off.

I dash out of the room and run full tilt boogie down the hallway to the Atrium, crying. *No no no no.* I slide up to the information desk and blubber my way through Steve's problems to a nice white-haired woman named Roberta, who is the epitome of patience. I hope I'm making sense. I tell her that Steve had a recent liver transplant, was doing well but then a few days ago deteriorated, and we don't know why but it might be from Prograf. I tell her that I ran into one of his former nurses on the transplant unit about an hour ago and told her what was going on with Steve and without hesitation, she said "That's Prograf."

Roberta makes no attempt to stop me. She's lasering in on me, assessing: dangerous/not dangerous? I might have looked a little crazy, but she stays with me, God bless her.

"I just can't get anyone to help us," I say in a rush. "We've been in the ER three times in as many days. If I don't get the help we need, I'm going to dial 911, I swear to God I am, and see if the police can get some answers. I need to reach Steve's transplant surgeon, Dr. Anthony, and have him come to the ER right now because he knows what Steve was like before the transplant. The difference is horrific. Can you help me reach his office?"

"Certainly," she says, all calm and dignified, and scans her directory, then dials.

Roberta reaches Dr. Anthony's assistant and hands me the phone. I explain everything. She says he's in surgery now, and can't come. In fact, none of the surgeons are available to come over right now.

"Fine." I slam down the phone.

Roberta very calmly and coolly says, "I'm so sorry you're having such trouble. Tell you what. Let me call the ombudsman. It's their job to help out with these things." She scans her directory again and dials. I'm convinced she believes I would actually call the police.

She's not wrong.

I nod, wiping my eyes, my cheeks, no doubt bearing a distinct resemblance to a raccoon. I've never been much of a make-a-fuss kind of gal. I never send restaurant meals back to the kitchen if they aren't "just right," never start fights with random strangers, and in the distant past have taken at face value what doctors have told me. But now? All those years of being a Nice Girl— trying to please, mostly others, not myself—have been upended. I'm finding out what I'm really made of: A shark-toothed adversary with Midwestern tomboy grit. Do *not* mess with me or someone I love, or with my metaphors.

I took on my Dad at 16—I sure as hell can take on these people!

Roberta hangs up and says, "I finally reached Janice. Follow me and I'll take you to her office." I start breathing again, hoping to dampen enough of my fury to string the words together. We walk quickly down the blue tiled hall.

When we arrive at the ombudsman's office, I say, "Thank you, Roberta, for helping me. You may have just saved a life."

"That's my job, dear," she says and pats my shoulder. "I hope everything works out OK for you and your husband."

Janice invites me to sit down. Through my tears, I launch into my story. When I finish, Janice scoots her chair back and says, "Just a minute. I'll be right back." I don't know if she's going to call the police on me or what.

She returns and says "There's a transplant surgeon on her way to the ER right now. I hope she can help you."

"Oh, my God, really? You did that? Thank you, thank you," I say. I spring out of the chair, leap out of her office in one giant step, cheetah through the atrium, wave at Roberta as I pass, do a jab step around others as I fly down the hall, make a wrong turn, oops, backtrack to the ER. Stop. Breathe. One thousand one, one thousand two, one thousand fucking three. I enter Steve's room.

Landon is talking with a short blond woman. I extend my hand to her and say, "Hi! I'm Rosie, Steve's wife. Thanks for coming. Has Landon filled you in on all the problems Steve has been having?" Her name tag says "Dr. Warner."

"Yes." I can't decide from her mien if she's concerned or not. And, if not, why the hell not? But I tell myself, *pissing her off is not going to help Steve, so shut it, Rosie.*

"You know," I say in my non-hysterical voice, "I was just on the transplant unit and ran into a couple of nurses who cared for Steve on his first admission. They told me that this is all down to Prograf! They said they never had problems when patients were put on Cyclosporine, so I would like him taken off Prograf and put on that."

She stiffens. "Well, it's possible." Thin, ungenerous lips.

"Possible? What else could it be? His CAT scan was fine, or so we were told. He has no history of mental illness, so what else in the world could be causing all this trouble? I want him off Prograf, can you do that?"

I'm losing control and can see that I'm pissing her off, but ask me if I care. "We've been told by other docs in the ER that Steve would get better on his own. Well, I'm here to tell you, that's not happening. He's only gotten worse and it's killing us trying to take care of him."

Dr. Warner says, "I need to consult with the surgeons who did the transplant, but I'll get back to you. In the meantime, we are going to admit Mr. West to the transplant unit until we can get this straightened out."

"Well, good. Thank you." I glance at Landon who is nodding his head in agreement.

But what if my Sweetheart is already too far gone?

Chapter Nineteen

Now What?

Monday, April 6, 2015
8:30 p.m.

S teve is being wheeled up to his new room on the transplant unit, with Landon and me hurrying behind. I don't know why hope is still sticking around. I'm back to square one in the hands of the very people who have ignored my concerns. But if all I have left is hope then by God, I'm gonna do whatever it takes to make hope dance to my tune, aren't I? To see to it that hope whispers in the ears of Steve's doctors to make them do the right thing: knock off the offending Prograf.

And give us a good explanation for why they have been allowing Steve and us to suffer.

But what if I'm wrong, what if nurses Karen and Sharon are wrong? What if it's not Prograf, but something else that the doctors are not telling us?

I have a right to know, whatever it is. But Karen and Sharon responded so quickly when I told them why we brought Steve to the ER, I doubt they're wrong. They have no reason to mislead me. They're the ones tasked with the daily care of liver transplant patients; so they should know.

Why should I, a lay person, be saddled with figuring this out? I do have some medical knowledge, thank God, but for heaven's sakes, I'm not a doctor, I'm not a nurse. Steve is depending on me to get him out of this hell hole. What if I can't? What if I'm making things worse?

I've got to get him out of here.

Steve's bed has been settled into position by his new nurse, Becky, who is kind and attentive. She's seen him before.

"Welcome, Mr. West. I'm sorry you had to come back, but it's still good to see you." She busies herself reading his online record.

Steve smiles. "Yes," he says, "they tell me I need a tune-up." His mentation has revived a bit, his sentence-making ability squeaking through.

"Well, you've come to the right place then."

She bustles around to set him up: oxygen, IV, BP, the usual. I ask her about his meds.

"Do you still see Prograf on the list?"

"Yes, ma'am, I do. The doctors will make their rounds in the morning, so you can talk to them about it at that time."

"OK, thanks." Landon and I exchange eye rolls.

I plop down next to him on the window seat.

"How are you doing," I say.

"I'm OK. I just want them to get rid of the Prograf, if that's what's causing Dad to act like a psycho."

I laugh. Steve, a psycho? This will make a funny story after he recovers, if he recovers.

Remember that time you lost your mind?

"Are you going to be able to stay with him all night, again?" I plead to Landon, trying not to plead, but I am so done, spent, drained, kaput.

"Sure. I've done this before." He points toward the plaid vinyl window seat. "I'll just pull off these seat pads onto the floor. They make a pretty decent bed."

"You're a godsend, Landon. I've got to go home and crash. I can't take much more."

I can see why some people go out, buy guns and shoot up the place. Something's gone terribly wrong, and they just can't take it anymore.

I need to sleep and putter around the apartment, get my quotidian on and go to Walmart. That seems like such a luxury right now. Who knew—Walmart, the quintessential destination for the broken ones? Steve needs some better-fitting clothes and some other items I cannot now recall. I have no idea of where any other stores might be, but Walmart is on my way to the apartment, so Walmart it is.

"Sure. That's fine. I've got this," says Landon as he gives me a hug.

"I'm so grateful that you could come and help out. He needs a lot more attention than one person can give. If the docs come in before I get here in the morning, and I'm sure they will, would you please ask them about Prograf? What are their plans for shit-canning it? You're a guy, maybe they will be more forthright with you. You never know."

"Sure, I'll be here," he says and smiles.

Steve sparks some alertness and says, "Where are you going?"

"Not far, Honey, but I've got to get some sleep tonight. Tomorrow morning I'm going to buy you some shirts and pants that fit. Can you think of anything else you need?"

"A new shaver." He says, the light inside still dim, but dim is better than dark.

"You got it. Landon is staying all night and you have your bunny so you should be fine. I'll be in around noon or so. Is that OK?" I lean over to give him a kiss.

"As long as I have my Dude."

On my way out, I tell the nurse that Landon is going to spend the night, and would she mind bringing him a pillow and some sheets and blankets?

"Sure," she says, "I'll be happy to." I've noticed that Landon, modest as he is about his looks, is honey for the worker bees. Maybe I should sic him on the female nurse practitioners and transplant surgeon about Prograf. Maybe he can get answers that I cannot.

11:30 p.m.

Home never felt so good. Fluffy arrives, wanting attention. I'm happy to oblige. "Hey, there, Fluffy, how're you doing, girl?" We think she's a girl, but it's hard to tell with all that fur. I deliver a few scritches, then say, "Would you like a late snack?" I've never met a cat who would say no, so I enter the apartment, head for the fridge and return outside with a can of Fancy Feast. "Here you go, Darling," I say as I spoon it into her bowl. Also top up her water bowl. "Night night, sweet kitty," I say as I move inside.

Oh, the silence. No troubled sounds of Steve perseverating on "Glucerna," no heartbreaking struggle to get him to eat or drink, no Landon pleading, "Come on Dad, one more bite?"

Silence. Complete empty, fragrant silence. My ears are ringing with it. My mouth is alive with its sweet taste. How weird is that?

I need a hot shower, a very long, long hot shower, under as much water as the city can supply. I want to store up memories of water abundance because my beloved California is still in drought.

I strip in my bedroom, reach for the robe, and scuff off to the bathroom, where I stay under the downpour longer than is probably good for the skin, prune-wrinkling and all, but I don't care. I linger under the watery pulsating salvation until I am rinsed with clarity, disabused of my fears. I step out onto the mat and dry myself with a fluffy white terry towel while humming my favorite Nanci Griffith tune, "Love at the Five and Dime."

Nanci describes a Woolworth's store as smelling like popcorn and chewing gum rubbed around on the bottom of a leather-soled shoe. Can't argue with that.

Whenever I hear Nanci singing that song, it ignites an old memory of my beloved mother, long since dead. I would love once more to sit next to her on a red vinyl stool at the Formica lunch counter at Woolworth's in Moline, and instead of waiting to find out if she could afford for me to have an entire sandwich, I would whip out a twenty and tell her, "Mom, let's have whatever we want."

How I loved that Woolworth's. For me, as a young teen going to the big city with Mom—don't know what for, didn't care, as long as I ended up sitting next to her at the Woolworth counter for a ham salad sandwich on white bread and a piece of cherry pie with a thick brown glazed crust, and even if we had to split it, it was closer to heaven than we Lutherans had a right to imagine.

Tuesday, April 7, 2015

I wake up at 8:00 a.m., somewhat refreshed, but not restored. I am profoundly wrecked by this experience, beginning with the horrific evaluation week and now Steve's deterioration. I'm not sure I'm ever going to escape from the deep, dark sewer of trauma I've been flushed into. I had assumed all along that moving here for Steve's transplant would be stressful, but this?

Seriously?

Terminally jaded, I try not to imagine the horror show that awaits.

Chapter Twenty

GASLIGHTING 101

Tuesday, April 7, 2015
10:30 a.m.

I guide our Kia Rio out into the misty rain, on my way to Walmart. I'm thrilled to be free—a grade schooler who's just been told, "No school! It's a snow day!" Time to hit the hills with our sleds or strap on our skates because the small-town roads are icy and skatable. Hot chocolate all around.

I'm not eager to phone Landon at the hospital to see about Steve. If anything bad has happened, Landon would have called me. I want to keep my brain and heart from being hijacked by Steve's medical catastrophe for as long as I can. I arrive at the parking lot and slide out of the car, turning my face to the glorious rain and scuttle inside.

I feel like Rip Van Winkle, free from liver trauma for the first time in months. Everything seems new and strange. I push the cart slowly up and down the aisles, looking here and there as if I'd never before seen such things: a shelf full of books; a stationery aisle with cards for every occasion, but none for a woman so worn out she has barely enough energy to sigh; stacks of cat food.

I'm glad to be among normal people, doing normal things. Just leisurely browsing for men's underwear, cotton shirts and sweat pants makes me giddy. I paw over the selection and find some items I think will fit and that Steve might like. If not, I can always return them to my Walmart Valhalla.

I wander the hardware aisle, one of my favorites, not that I'm particularly handy, but if I were, I would buy tons of stuff. Just think of all the things you can fix with these just-right items. There's a solution for everything, all except for my honey's deterioration and my despair.

In the personal grooming aisle, I find the shaver Steve needs to spruce himself up.

After sating my wanderlust while dreaming and dissociating, I search for the check-out counter with the longest line so I can read the *National Enquirer* without buying it. The clerk is friendly and efficient, and soon I am on my way.

I call Landon from the car, tell him I'll be there in about twenty minutes, and ask,

"What's up?"

"Dad spent the entire night moaning."

"What? Moaning? Was he in pain or something?"

Oh, God, now what?

"The nurse checked him out and there didn't seem to be anything wrong. He is still crazy—mumbling, not making sense."

"Did the doc come in and say anything about discontinuing Prograf?"

"I asked, but when I brought up the subject, he got kind of vague; so no, I never got a concrete answer about when or if Dad would be taken off it. Same thing when a nurse practitioner stopped by. It's all very mysterious."

"Oh, crap. I tell you what. As soon as I get there, why don't you take the car and go back to the apartment and get some rest. Could you stay with him again tonight?"

"Sure."

Who do I have to call to get a straight answer? A transplant coordinator? *Ha.* Coordinators around here are like cockroaches. As soon as you shine a light on them, they scurry under the woodwork. They should hire me to design a new system. Easy Peasy. One transplant coordinator assigned to, say, no more than three patients and their families, from beginning to end. The family would know then exactly whom to turn to for questions or problems.

But, I guess if they are firm in their decision to withhold information from patients and families, it wouldn't matter what system they had. You would still be left in the dark.

Imagine how much heartache I would have been spared, though, if such a system had been in place and if the person had been willing to tell us the truth.

I pull into the hospital parking lot, remove my catch o'the day nestled in my Walmart bags, strap on my fanny pack, grip my tote and prepare for . . . for whatever.

When I arrive at Steve's room, he is dozing, but I plant a kiss on his cheek anyway and say, "I'm baaack. And, I've got some loot for you." I wave the Walmart bags in the air. He stirs to life.

I hand Landon the car keys and say, "I hope you get a nice, long nap!"

"Me, too," he says and pockets the keys. "Did you park in the usual spot?"

"Yes," I say, and give him a hug.

OK, well, then, see you guys later. Bye, Dad," he says and gives Steve a peck on the forehead. Be good."

He trudges out the door.

"OK, Dude. See you later," says Steve. "Thanks for everything, man."

"A young, dark-haired nurse practitioner named Jacob enters Steve's room.

"How're we doing today, Mr. West?" Why do they insist on using the royal *we*? An old joke has it that the only people qualified to use the royal *we* are emperors, editors and those with a tapeworm.

"Fine," Steve says with good cheer. I don't know how he does it. Good cheer hasn't knocked on my door in months.

I know that if I don't speak up right now, I will be ignored. It's as if I, the caretaker, am only here for Steve's amusement, not for relieving them of the trouble of saving his life. I'm aware that I am jaded and cranky, can hear it in my own voice, and wish it were not so.

"He's not fine, Jacob. Have you read his chart? About how out of it he's been—his word salad, his inability to swallow his pills, his—"

"Yes, I have," he says and casts a glance my way but without seeing me.

"Well, then, are you going to switch him from Prograf to Cyclosporine? I've been told by two nurses that Steve's behavior is all down to Prograf."

"Well, we're looking at that."

Why won't she just shut up, I can hear him thinking. *Who does she think she is?*

"Well, would you like to *actually* look at it?" I say and walk toward him. "I've got a video here of Steve at home trying to walk with his walker down the hall after his Prograf was increased. And another video of him in full word salad mode. Those will show you everything you need to know."

I reach for my phone and start scrolling through the videos.

"No, that's all right. I think I've got the picture," he says and backs away.

Yeah, but I'm thinking *you don't know jack.*

Your choices are a) to scold him for not listening to you, or b) to shut up. You choose the latter. The power dynamics regarding Steve's care have been made clear. Doctors are in charge and do not wish to be questioned, especially by wives or nurses.

★★★

According to Dr. Paige L. Sweet, sociologist at Harvard University, gaslighting is a gendered phenomenon and rooted in social inequalities.

Well, how much more unequal can you get than when you are in the hands of a doctor? Unless he or she is a remarkable exception? I couldn't help but wonder if Landon had been alone and in charge of Steve's care, would they be dismissing him in the same way they are dismissing me now — ignoring his pleas when he offers to show them the videos? No way to know.

In "The Sociology of Gaslighting," Dr. Sweet notes that "Gaslighting . . . is primarily a sociological rather than psychological phenomenon."[2]

In the eponymous movie, Charles Boyer works to convince Ingrid Bergman that she is insane so he can take over her estate. How does he do this? Among other things, he alternately dims and brightens the house gaslights, and when she asks him about this, he convinces her, the poor dear, that her imagination is playing tricks on her and that she's going crazy. She begins to believe him. After all, he's the man of the house, she, just the little woman. Being gaslit is entirely familiar to Bergman's character. It does not occur to her to challenge Boyer.

Dr. Sweet points out that the tactics used (most often by men against women) are gendered in that they rely on the association of femininity with irrationality: "You're too emotional. "You're crazy." "You don't know what you're talking about." "You made me do it." "You're not thinking correctly," and so on.

Thus, to be female, is to be irrational.

Where have we heard that before?

Women have, of course, been dismissed and disrespected for eons; nothing new about that. It's an age-old sport.

But one man stands out for the impact he's had on the status of women.

Sigmund Freud.

Freud developed his theories, or rather his shameless lies, about women in 19th century Vienna.

Women, at that time, were treated as little more than the property of their husbands. They had no agency, no power or control over their own lives. Domestic duties, but not politics or education or employment, were the only things open to them. They were confined to child rearing and taking care of their husbands.

During the initial days when Freud was developing his theories and the practice of psychoanalysis, he attracted and treated many women. In their sessions with Freud, they often confided in him that they had been sexually abused by their fathers and/or other adult males when they were children.

He believed them.

He also believed that such early abuse was a contributing factor to their current problems, often labeled in those days as "hysteria."

Freud even wrote up his findings in a paper, entitled, "The Aetiology of Hysteria," which he presented before the Society for Psychiatry and Neurology, Vienna, April 21, 1896:

" . . . I therefore put forward the thesis that at the bottom of every case of hysteria there are one or more occurrences of premature sexual experience, occurrences which belong to the earliest years of childhood but which can be reproduced through the work of psycho-analysis in spite of the intervening decades."[3]

In other words, Freud was telling his mostly male audience the truth: his clients had been sexually abused by their fathers and/or other adult males when they were children, and that those horrendous events provided some of the underpinning for their illnesses as adults.

The male physicians in his audience were outraged. Who knows, perhaps many were themselves abusers. (Current statistics reveal that one out of every three women have been sexually abused. And those are just the ones we know about.)

Freud was so worried about being shunned by his colleagues and afraid of losing their referrals that he committed the unforgiveable sin—betraying those women and forever after rendering the stories of all girls and women suspect.

Instead of sacking up and standing behind his research and backing the women who had trusted and confided in him, he took the coward's way out and altered his theory, i.e. altered their truths to save his financial and professional skin.

He then claimed that, oops, he'd made a mistake. He suddenly realized that their sexual abuse had not actually happened, but in fact was only a product of their distorted imaginings.

This was a theory he could sell to his colleagues, one they were happy to receive, one that took them off the hook for their own crimes.

But in that fatal moment, Freud threw women under the bus for generations to come.

In that moment, he mainlined into western civilization, the belief that, at their core, women were fantasists, not to be trusted and that his patients' memories of seduction and rape were in fact just that—fantasies, arising from the minds of irrational women.

It was easy for him to do—women had no power, he was the great Dr. Freud, and who were they to question him?

Out of his own deep cowardice, he, a priori, branded women with ignominy for all time: women were not reliable; women were prone to lying; women couldn't be trusted.

Anita Hill? Christine Blasey Ford? Every other victim of sexual abuse who dares to come forward?

Consider how easily Dr. Larry Nasser convinced young female gymnasts that his abuse was not really abuse but, rather, standard treatment. After all, he was the trusted authority who had been using his vaginal and anal penetrative treatment on them for years and getting away with it.

Nasser is now rotting in jail for the rest of his life, but the trauma he inflicted on those girls lives on in the women they have become. And in the lives of parents who were sometimes present in the room when their daughters were being abused.

How easy it is, even now, to put women on their back foot by telling them they don't know what they're talking about. The Me Too movement is a step in the right direction, but will it go far enough?

I don't believe that Steve's doctors and nurses deliberately set out to harm him or Landon and me, but that was the undeniable result of their withholding the truth. They were so intent on keeping him on Prograf, that we and our concerns and complaints had been rendered, for lack of a better word, invisible. It's as if we had opened our mouths, but nothing of our concerns reached their ears or their hearts.

No one showed any concern or curiosity. No one paid attention to us. Our insurance company had to pay for our three unnecessary trips to the emergency room—a lot of money down the drain.

So, how were we supposed to feel? Confused? Angry? Scared to death? Some might like to quibble with the use of the word gaslighting, but the facts seem clear: they were deliberately withholding information.

Hippocrates, whose oath all physicians must take to "First Do No Harm," would not have approved.

Chapter Twenty-One

Is This the Way Our World Ends?

Wednesday, April 8, 2015
10:00 a.m.

Hoping against hope for a miracle while wondering what lunacy awaits us today, I enter Steve's room. Landon once again has stayed all night with Steve. I hand over the car keys as soon as I arrive and thank him. I'm beyond grateful. Couldn't wait to scarper last night.

Word salad is not an attractive feature in a partner. Nothing you'd want to include on your Tinder profile: "Looking for a crazy man who talks in fruits and vegetables; needs constant caretaking with no fear that he'll ever be normal."

I'm not proud of feeling abandoned and testy about not having my fully functioning partner returned to me. It's strange how our roles have been upended. Me, caretaker, him child. Will he ever be normal again? Assuming that Prograf is the cause of this crazy quilt, what kind of damage is it doing to his brain from which he might never recover? And if it isn't Prograf, why am I not hearing about that? Why the radio silence? They've done an MRI, CAT scans and EEG's, all supposedly normal.

So what's left?

***

When I was the Coordinator of an out-patient head injury program, I developed uncharacteristic patience with those young men and women whose brains had been scrambled: diving accidents, car accidents, motorcycle run-ins, gunshot wounds. In spite of their short-term memory problems, their difficulties with impulse control, reasoning and planning, their senses of humor remained intact.

Where in the brain does humor reside?

One afternoon, one of my higher-functioning patients, 23-year-old Don Sinclair, wheeled himself into my office for help in completing a form. Though severely injured in a car accident two years prior, Don lived semi-independently. Despite his severe dysarthria (weakness in the muscles used for speech, resulting in slowed and sometimes unintelligible sounds), I could still understand him.

When he asked if I would help him, I said, "Sure, Don, that's the least I could do."

He smiled, rolled his wheelchair closer, leaned toward me and said, with a twinkle in his sharp eyes, "What's . . . the . . . most . . . you . . . could . . . do . . . Rosie?"

We laughed so loudly that one of my co-workers stopped by to see what the fun was all about.

I enjoyed being someone the patients could count on. All the same, I knew how lucky I was to be able to go home at the end of the day. Their families, most often mothers, were stuck forever with their adult child-like children. I looked on with sadness, watching them become more and more bedraggled as the realization rolled in that their son or daughter would never fully recover.

All their hopes and dreams for their beloved had vanished during one split second of someone's bad judgment.

★★★

But here we are again on the transplant unit where time climbs into the wrong end of a telescope. Forever shuttled between the wide angle and the narrow focus, the days blur together, and clarity seems forever out of view.

On one end, we have Word Salad Steve, and on the other, Rosie the Rescuer, or rather Rosie the Ersatz Rescuer. The jury is still out on whether or not she will succeed.

The morning train of doctors and nurse practitioners rolls in around 10:30. One by one, they hop off for brief stops but do not deliver the answers we need. Overall, they seem pleased with Steve's recovery, except for the crazy thing.

If they know something I don't know, I wish they would tell me. I'm weary of asking and not receiving answers. I'm aware that I'm morphing into zombie land, walking and talking but with little vibrancy of affect. I know he needs caretaking. I need it, too, but that's not on the agenda for now. I'm hanging in until the day when Steve and I, as equals, can laugh about the madness we survived during his transplant.

But will that day ever come? And, if so, when?

I perch on the edge of Steve's bed and attempt to talk to him. His conversations are so convoluted and nonsensical that there's no place to insert a comment. He's afraid of "massive propellers in the basement whirling round and round to destroy the hospital." I have no choice but to play along with him. "Is that right?" "Well, whaddya make of that?" Or, "That sounds scary."

No sense saying, "What the hell are you talking about? I'm pretty sure there are no propellers in the basement." It's likely he can twig to my disingenuousness, but I give it my best shot. That's all I've got, even though I know it's inadequate.

No matter what I do, I'm always going to feel guilty because it's never enough and resentful because it's never enough. But this is not about me.

Anna, his nurse, cranks Steve's bed up to sitting position so I can I tackle his meds. He must have his medications on time, and I tell her that maybe I can help. I don't know how these nurses do their jobs day after day after day with, for the most part, patience and kindness. I know she has other tasks to accomplish. I watched as she grew frustrated when trying to give Steve his pills. With our cat Billy, I use a piller device to give him his asthma medication. But then, Billy is not crazy. He holds still while I pill him. Too bad there's not a piller for humans.

"Here's the deal, Steve," I say. "I know you're worried about propellers, but they are not here yet. So, in the meantime, how about you take your anti-rejection pills—you know the ones that keep your body from rejecting your shiny new liver? And you need some food, too. You've lost sixty pounds, and it would be good if we can help you put some of that back on."

"Yes," he says and sounds convincing until I bring one pill to his mouth and ask him to open up. He doesn't.

I say, "That's good, Steve. That's a start. Now, can you open your mouth?"

I want to be anywhere but here.

He nods, looking like a normal, though very skinny human in a fresh gown after Anna assisted him in the shower this morning before I arrived and applied his new shaver to his days-old stubble. She is not put off by his crazy, because, unlike some other patients, at least up until now, he's not been a mean crazy, just a sweet addled crazy.

I open my mouth to demonstrate.

"Can you do this?" I say, slowly opening and shutting my mouth. I open my mouth again and hold the pill near my tongue, working on the theory of "monkey-see-monkey-do."

He lowers his jaw just enough so I can insert the pill.

"Now, can you close your mouth?" I move my hand under his jaw and gently urge it upward. Success!

"Next, let's have some Glucerna to help you swallow and get that pill down there where it can do some good, OK? The only reason you're having such a problem now is the drugs; it's not you, Sweetheart, but right now, I need you to do what I ask you to. The sooner we can lick this problem, the sooner we can go home." I can tell I have punched a small hole through the mist. He nods.

"Glucerna."

Two hours, eleven pills, one Glucerna, three-quarters of a banana and a tangerine later, success!

About 4:00 p.m., a new nurse arrives with two student nurses in tow and asks if they could interview Steve. Steve does enjoy an audience and initially seems to appreciate their questions, which he answers in word salad. He seems fine with them, up until he isn't. He becomes more and more agitated by their presence, grunting and squirming around in the bed, and I have to ask them to leave.

"So now you know what can happen to a patient on the transplant unit," I say to them on their way out the door. In their minds, they have probably crossed off transplant from their list of desired rotations.

Once again, Anna attempts to give Steve his late afternoon pills, and Steve resists. I say I'd be happy to help out again. She seems glad for the relief. Even though Steve balks at every damn pill I want to give him, when finally there are none left, he wants "one more, one more," and twists and grunts when I won't give him one more.

Explaining my reasons at this point is useless. Might as well try to convince a cat that the trip to the vet is for his own good. Seriously? Hiss, meow, scratch.

Steve begins to holler about the propellers in the basement. "They are going to come up through the floor and kill us all!" I inch away and say, "Steve, I need to go out into the waiting room and email our friends and family. They like to keep up with what's going on."

"No! You can stay here and use that computer," he growls, pointing to the one the nurses use. Then he hits my arm. This is not like Steve, but his eyes are wild.

I nudge further away. "Honey, I can't use that computer, that's for the nurses." Will the crazy never cease?

"Go out into the hall, find five nurses and hit them!"

That does it. Whatever shred of patience I have been ferociously hanging onto slips through my fingers like so many pieces of a jigsaw puzzle. I know I should have just gone along with him and said, "Sure, I'll do that," but my irritation is getting the best of me, and I say, with uncharacteristic force, "No, I'm not going to do that." He reaches forward and hits my arm again.

That is definitely not my Steve—a heinous dopplegänger has obviously kidnapped the original.

I strap on my fanny pack, hoist my tote bag and leave. I wave to Anna who has been watching from the glass-boothed section in Steve's room. It's an observational feature for patients such as Steve, who need constant monitoring and attention. I tell her I'll be in the waiting room if she needs me.

I know this is not my Steve, but I can't help being furious with him for hitting me. I sit down at the computer and update family and friends. I had been hoping for better news to share. I thank them on Steve's behalf for all the cards and letters and gifts. Just knowing we have people back home who are rooting for us has been a great comfort. They'd be horrified if they could see Steve in his current state. I promised to take good care of him.

How's that working out for you, Rosie?

I plop down in one of the seats and toss my bag onto its neighbor. I watch as some family members pace up and down the hall while others cluster together and speak in hushed tones, some wiping their eyes—each of us struggling in our own private hell.

Landon will be returning soon for the evening shift. Maybe he can get through to Steve. In the meantime, I do my best to lie down, contorting myself around the middle arm rest, using my tote bag as a pillow.

I've not long to rest before Anna flies down the hall toward me. I sit up. This is not going to be a friendly chat.

"Please, can you come back to the room?" she cries, with panic in her eyes. "Steve is very angry. He had a fit and threw the urine bottle all over the room, and I can't calm him down!"

"Oh, I'm s-so sorry," I stammer, trying to picture what she just described. "I don't know what I can do, but I'll try."

I leap up and follow her to the room. I move slowly toward Steve, intending to calm him, but he hollers, "Go away, go away," and strikes out at me. I leave the room and talk to Anna who has returned to the booth. She tells me she has put in a call to his transplant surgeon. Finally.

When I return to the room fifteen minutes later, I say nothing to Steve as I take over the window seat. Landon calls to tell me he's in the parking lot. He's ready to stay the night.

"Change of plans, Landon. Your Dad has gone bat crap crazy. I need to stay for a while longer; so could you just park the car and come on up? Maybe he'll calm down with you here."

I meet Landon hurrying down the hall and fill him in on Steve's psychotic behavior. "I'll stay outside of his room here while you go in to see if you can get through to him."

I watch as he cautiously approaches Steve, saying softly, "Dad, Dad, what's going on?"

Steve shakes his head; no words come out. I edge back into the waiting room. Observing Steve in this condition pains my heart.

About ten minutes later, Landon, walking slowly, with defeat etched on his handsome face, comes over and says, "Dad is just curled up at the end of the bed, staring, saying nothing. What is going on?"

"I'm so sorry. Maybe give him a few minutes alone and then go back in? I only seem to agitate him."

We wait another ten minutes. I trail behind Landon as he returns to the room. We notice Steve struggling to get out of bed.

"Hey, Dad, you need to go to the bathroom?" Landon says and rushes over to him.

Steve grunts. I hang back.

Landon stands at the end of the bed, waiting as usual for Steve to rise up so he can guide him to the bathroom.

Steve pushes off as if to stand, but in the next nanosecond he shoves Landon hard, pivots violently to his left, and dives down to the floor near the sink, lands on his knees, grabs the hard thick vertical panel fastened to the sink frame, yanks it off its steel bolts and slams it into his forehead with enough force to fracture his skull. I scream, Anna screams and hits the emergency button. Landon hollers and moves to help him, but before he can even reach Steve, two tall muscular young men appear—fruit fly fast—carrying soft restraints.

They move slowly toward Steve and bend down. "Mr. West, we're here to help. Are you OK?"

Steve lies on the floor, unmoving and silent.

I scream, "Don't hurt him, please don't hurt him!"

I can't hide my sobbing. Restraints? What the—

"We will be very careful, ma'am. We've done this many times before when a patient has had a meltdown." They could be twins, these handsome twenty-somethings, dressed in their blue scrubs, with short brown hair and bountiful muscles.

They reach out to Steve, who by now is calm and doesn't struggle. They carefully guide him up and toward the bed, saying, "We want to get you back to bed so you're safe."

They help him slide into bed. They hold out the soft blue restraints and tell him, "We're just going to tie these loosely around your wrists so that you don't hurt yourself. Is that OK, Mr. West?"

Steve looks around, nods and smiles, as if he's happy to be where he is.

Landon and I stand dazed and speechless, awaiting the next volley.

Thinking of T.S. Elliott, I wonder, *Is this the way your world ends, is this the way your world ends, is this the way your world ends, not with a whimper but a bang?*

Chapter Twenty-Two

AFTERSHOCKS

Wednesday, April 8, 2015
11:00 p.m.

I'm standing in Steve's room, a statue, barely breathing, holding onto the back of a chair, wobbly, as though we'd been shaken up by an earthquake. Gobsmacked, I sit down, waiting for the aftershock, incredulous about what I have just witnessed. I watch the nurses tend to Steve who's now as calm as a baby lamb. I glance over at Landon, slumping on the window seat, soft tears in his eyes. How horrible this must be to see his dad in a psychotic state and in restraints.

I've nothing to offer anyone right now.

I badly need a very long, hot shower to cleanse and calm my beleaguered spirit.

Anna summons me out into the hall to meet with Dr. Warner, the wispy blond transplant surgeon I met in the ER a few days ago. I feel grubby and disheveled in her presence. I notice several other people slow-walking near Steve's room, trying not to gawk but gawking nonetheless to see what the fuss was all about.

Nothing to see here, folks, just another near-fatal crack-up.

Dr. Warner wants my approval to give Steve Haldol. Haldol is a powerful anti-psychotic drug, often used in nursing homes to keep patients sedated and quiet.

This is the first time anyone has asked my permission for anything.

My reaction is swift and feral, no time for a breath. "No! I know what Haldol is. I'm afraid that might make him crazier than he is, if that's even possible. He's been using Restoril at home on occasion to help him sleep. Can we use that?"

Dr. Warner, shorter than me by about five inches, looks up and says, "That should be fine." I'm surprised she is not going to fight me. It's late. Maybe she just wants to go home to her non-psychotic family. Can't blame her. The life of a transplant surgeon can't be easy. So many ways for a patient to go south, to wit, Steve's psychotic meltdown.

Anna, the petite brunette who has been Steve's favorite nurse thus far, says, furrowing her brow, "But Restoril is not available in the hospital formulary." I adore her for being so kind to Steve during the worst of his word salad days.

"Oh for Pete's sake," I sigh and glance from one to the other. "I know Steve brought some with him. Could we go get that and use it tonight?"

Dr. Warner says, "Yes. That should be OK." Again, no fuss. Do I look so feral that she wants to get away from me as soon as she can?

"Thanks," I say and whirl back to the room to ask Landon if he would please head to the apartment and scour Steve's dopp kit for the bottle of Restoril. I yank my keys out of my fanny pack and hand them over.

I return to the hallway where Dr. Warner and Anna are talking softly.

Dr. Warner says, flatly, to me, "We're discontinuing his Prograf and putting him on Cyclosporine."

Under ordinary circumstances I'd feel admiration for any woman who succeeds in a field saturated with men. It can't have been easy. But as it is, whatever scintilla of regard I might have had for her drowns in her casual comment about trading in Prograf for Cyclosporine, with no accompanying acknowledgment of or apology for all the terror we've experienced.

That's like a new car dealer telling you, after your purchase six months ago, that, "We're going to give you a new set of tires because the ones that originally came with your car were crap and you found us out. Otherwise, we'd have been happy to let you keep driving on faulty treads."

I don't know whether to laugh or cry or punch Dr. Warner in the mouth. It took Steve giving himself a possible fractured skull or at least a concussion for her to make that decision? And now we're supposed to be grateful?

Astonishment is too cheap a word.

I opt for being nice. No sense launching a grenade at the moment.

But I'm on a roll. "I'd like Steve to have a CAT scan as soon as possible," I say. "To make sure he hasn't fractured his skull or anything. Can you do that, please?"

"Sure," she says with no reluctance. Upon closer inspection, she looks beat herself.

Goodness knows how many transplant surgeries she has performed today.

I thank her for coming tonight to learn for herself how Steve has been suffering. And how Landon and I have been suffering. What I don't hear is a confession that all along his doctors knew that Prograf was the culprit and for crazy reasons of their own, decided not to tell us. We might never know why.

I could kick myself for not doing my own research at the time. If I had done, I might have discovered some answers in the research articles I found much later at home.

When I Googled "Patients with bad reactions to Prograf," I found several articles—1994[4], 2009[5], 2011[6], 2013[7]— well before 2015 when Steve received his transplant. All the articles described patients who experienced the exact same symptoms Steve had shown after his Prograf was increased.

There was even an official diagnosis, "akinetic mutism."[8]

They had to have known about this. Karen and Sharon had seen this condition before. How hard would it have been for his doctors to tell us? They clearly knew, yet withheld the information.

There's no forgiveness for that.

I utter a weak "Thank you."

"Certainly," she says, shakes my hand and hastens down the hallway.

Landon returns with Steve's Restoril. We give him one capsule and soon Steve is out like the battered nut job that he is.

I tell Landon that Dr. Warner is discontinuing the Prograf and starting Cyclosporine.

"About time." He has changed his departure date, and now will leave on Tuesday, the 14th. That gives Steve a few more days to get sane and more fit.

If only.

We return to Steve's room. He's sleeping, gently snoring, blissfully unaware of all the chaos he's caused. Not his fault, of course. I thank Landon for the umpteenth time, and say good-night.

Thursday, April 9, 2015

The Greek god Morpheus lulls me to sleep around 2:00 a.m. I had told Landon before I left the hospital that I wouldn't be in until noon today. That I needed to decompress from last night's horror show. I've only been put through a wringer like this two other times, both at this hospital.

Once during Steve's evaluation when the surgical resident in the ER almost gave him heparin despite Steve's low platelet count and the other time a few days ago in the ER when Steve had a couple of seizures, and I had to threaten to call the police to get someone to help him. I hope never again to have my limits tested so severely.

The phone rings at 8:30 a.m. Oh, what fresh hell is this? It's Eric, the transplant pharmacist I met weeks ago when I attended his meeting with family members to learn all about the meds that transplant patients would be given. Funny, nothing was said about the potential side effects of Prograf during that meeting.

I'm pissed. Why didn't I think to call him as soon as Steve went crazy? He's a pharmacist. He'd have been the logical choice to ask. I've been letting Steve and Landon and myself down.

How could I have been so stupid?

Eric says, "I'd like to meet with you this morning about what happened last night. Can you be here by 10:30?"

How could I say no after all the fuss I've made? And, besides, he was damn cute, and I could use a bit more cute in my life right now. He's also extremely bright and knowledgeable; all in all, a very nice package.

"Sure. Where shall we meet?"

"I'll come to Mr. West's room at 10:30." I think about Eric's nice tight buns and how all the nurses are after him. Who will he end up with? Mary? Susan? Jack? Stay tuned to *As the Transplant Unit Turns.*

"Fine. Thanks," I say and dash to the shower, then to the kitchen for some quick eggs and toast and grab some snacks for later. I had hoped to sleep in at least until noon. But, duty calls.

I call Landon, who stayed overnight again with Steve. Steve is doing remarkably better today, after having slept well. He even ate his entire breakfast (!) without prompting. Hallelujah!

I arrive around 10:00 a.m. I tell Landon that Eric is stopping by at 10:30, and he's welcome to stay while I talk with him.

"I think you can handle this," he says and takes the keys. "I need some sleep. See you later."

Eric arrives spot on time. Steve is napping, and I don't want to wake him, so I talk with Eric in the hallway. He looks fresher than fresh. How does he do it?

"I understand Mr. West had a very bad night last night," he says, leaning close.

"Yes, you could say that."

"I'm recommending we put Mr. West on Seroquel at night," he says. "That's a better drug for him right now than Restoril." Flashing brown eyes, sturdy shoulders.

"Isn't that also an anti-psychotic? Dr. Warner wanted to put him on Haldol last night and I said no. Why would Seroquel be better for him?"

Please make me believe you.

"We use it all the time on the unit. It calms patients down and helps them get a good night's sleep, which is so important for their recovery."

Eric is very convincing, but just the thought of an anti-psychotic worries me. I also know that benzodiazepines such as Restoril can be addictive and that's not a good thing. Eric is so endearing and smart and dedicated that I let my guard down.

"OK. Let's do that, but can you give him the minimum dose at first to see how he does?"

"Absolutely. We will start it tonight."

If Eric had asked me to run away with him to Santorini, I might have done. Anything to get out of this liver hell. I don't want to be responsible for Steve anymore. I want to collapse into the arms of this kind caring man and hear him say, "There, there, my darling, everything is going to be fine. Just leave it to me."

Sunday, April 12, 2015
10:00 a.m.

Steve has been doing better and better the past three days, off the Prograf and on the Cyclosporine. Karen and Sharon, the nurses I encountered over a week ago were correct.

Prograf makes some patients go nuts.

Eric was right about Seroquel. Landon, who continues to spend the nights with Steve, tells me Steve is sleeping better than ever and that most of his word salad has retreated to whatever garden from whence it came. There might be a stray leaf of radicchio turning up now and again, but mostly we've arrived at a salad-free zone. He is now sitting up in his chair, looking pretty chipper, his robe pulled tight over his hospital gown, his feet snug in his pressure socks and slippers.

I know I should have blasted every doctor and nurse who had ignored me about Steve's reaction to Prograf, and lodged a complaint to the hospital CEO and the Joint Commission for Hospital Accreditation. But we're not on the home stretch yet.

So best to keep my head down, my mouth shut and hope like hell that no more bad things happen.

I say my usual thanks and good-bye to Landon who is headed back to the apartment to sleep. Thank God he doesn't have to leave for another two days. I want Steve to have enough time to recover and be more independent with me at the apartment.

Steve says, "Thanks, Dude. See you tonight." Landon tosses a wave.

I sit down on the green plaid vinyl window seat near Steve. "Welcome back, Sweetheart," and give him a big smacker on his cheek. "It's nice to see the real you again!"

"I feel fine," he says and leans up to kiss me. His beautiful brown eyes are once again tracking his smile. Someone is actually home behind them now.

"You were quite the show, the other night, you know that?"

"I just couldn't get anyone to listen to me. Not the CIA, the FBI, the nurses, you or anyone. I was convinced that those propellers were coming up from the basement to kill all of us. I thought maybe I could hide under the sink."

"I'm surprised you remember all that. How's your head?" I say and examine the welt on his forehead.

"Fine. It's only a bit tender."

"Have they given you a CAT scan yet?"

"No. I had an amazing dream last night. I dreamt that I was in the boxing ring with the Grim Reaper. When the bell clanged, I charged forward to the middle of the mat and clobbered him hard with my fist on the top of his head. He exploded lickety-split, and his ashes collapsed violently into a heap, with his scythe landing on top of the pile."

"Whoa! That'll teach him to mess with my sweetheart!" Steve has always had a very sturdy spirit. Not even the Grim Reaper was gonna bring him down.

"Damn straight."

"Nobody's going to take you out!" I laugh now at the memory of what he did. Though skinny, with a gaunt face and flaccid arms, he's still strong enough to yank a ¾" laminated plywood board from its steel bolts and hit himself in the head with it.

Who does that?

His doctors are tinkering with his medications, searching for the proper balance. His white count has dipped a bit so they are giving him something to increase it. All in all, it's very tricky business to keep his immune system from rejecting his liver, while at the same time making sure they don't suppress it so much that it is no longer able to snuff out the usual attackers—colds, flus and other assorted viral and bacterial infections.

Steve is receiving physical and occupational therapy again and can now follow three-step commands: "Put on your robe, put on your slippers and stand up by your walker."

An impossibility during the days of words and salad.

Steve has been doing so well that the staff are making noises about discharging him. That sets off alarm bells. It's one thing for Steve to be able to walk safely up and down a smooth hallway for a few yards with a physical therapist by his side; it's another for him to be independent in the apartment with me. He needs to be able to transfer into and out of the car by himself, fold up the walker, put it into the trunk and take it out again, go to the bathroom without help and other assorted ADL's (Activities of Daily Living.)

With Landon soon leaving, it's all going to be down to me. I've spoken to the physical therapist, the nurse, and the nurse practitioner about this, telling them I'd like Steve to go to an in-patient rehabilitation unit for a few days to improve his functioning. I mention that I'm not capable, that I'm still in a lot of pain from an old car accident and surgeries. I do not have enough upper body strength to catch him if he should fall. I'm aware that I look like a normal person, so I'm not sure they believe me. They say they will follow up with our health plan.

I've yet to hear from a social worker, the one person tasked specifically with helping families set up discharge plans. In my experience, the social worker always meets with the family soon after admission to establish a discharge plan so that the therapists can tailor their treatment plans accordingly. Ah, silly me. That would have been too sensible.

One day I'm told that Steve will be able to go to in-patient rehab. Relief. A few days later the answer is no. Fuck. I am aware that I have a right to refuse discharge from this hospital, but I refrain. I do not want them taking their pique with me out on him.

For a hospital eager to discharge Steve, no physical therapist has appeared for the past two days to walk him. I do it myself. So far so good. He is also doing his chair exercises.

"I need you to be as strong as possible," I tell him, "because it doesn't look like you're going to rehab."

In the meantime, a physician, a nurse practitioner and a social worker breeze into the room to talk with Steve and review his chart. Then they say that in-patient rehab would be authorized for Steve.

What?

"Wait a minute," I say, just as they turn to breeze back out again. "What about a plan for when he comes home? What about a list of resources for us, in case I need to contact someone to come in and help us?" Shirley, the social worker, says she'll return with a list for me.

Wednesday, April 14, 2015
9:00 a.m.

I've been waiting for the social worker to bring the information she promised and for Eric to show up to tell me that Walgreens is all set up with Steve's meds.

Fed up, I finally leave around 1:30 p.m. for a trip to Walgreens. By then, Landon had already taxied to the airport. I hated to say good-bye, but I knew he must go. He and Steve shared some teary moments before he left. I hugged him as he headed out the door and said, "You have no idea how much your help has meant to me, to us!"

"Oh, I think I have some idea. Keep me posted." My heart lurched as he left the room. Now I had no one to count on. He'd been shouldering all the physical burdens that I could not and still cannot handle.

I receive a call from Kelly, a rather careless twenty-something. Not Steve's favorite nurse, always acting put out whenever Steve asks for help with anything. "I thought you said you wanted to take him home today."

Oh, so now you care? In fact, I did not want to take him home to the apartment, but in-patient rehab has been taken off the table and I don't have enough fight left in me to protest.

Not gonna take the bait. Instead, I say, "When will he be ready?"

"Three or four or so."

"Thanks," I say and hang up. I'm at Walgreens to pick up Steve's meds. Bruce the pharmacist says there's a problem with Cyclosporine, because their record shows Steve is still on Prograf.

"No, he isn't," I say. "They had to discontinue Prograf because it made him crazy."

"I'll try to reach his doctor again," Bruce says. "I'll call you once I hear."

"Thanks."

I return to the apartment and call our Home Care agency to get referrals for a nurse's assistant to come and stay with us, if need be. They give me the names of several other agencies.

I call one to get their rates. More reasonable than I expected.

I call Steve to tell him I'm on my way back to the hospital. He answers right away. I hear Shirley, the social worker, in the background asking him if he'd received the pamphlets she left.

"No, I was in the bathroom."

"Well," she says, testily, "I left them. *Where are they*?" You'd have thought that at the very least, the social worker would be filled with the milk of human kindness, would you not?

Steve says to me, "Just a minute, Rosie. Shirley's here and wants me to find the information she said she left." I can hear him fumbling around. He finally locates them and shows them to Shirley.

Upon hearing this, she hustles out of the room.

"Nothing like full concierge service," I say to Steve. "I'll be there soon to pick you up and take you home to the apartment."

I return to the hospital around 3:30. I see no evidence that they are getting him ready to leave. Steve is still in his gown and still sporting bandages that should have come off days ago. I ask Kelly about this.

She says nothing, just sighs as she approaches Steve and starts to remove them. Steve winces when she starts to rip them off. His skin is very sensitive, and he asks if she can use some rubbing alcohol so that it won't hurt so much.

"We don't have any here," she says with barely contained irritation. "I'll have to go get some."

Shirley calls to find out if I got the info she'd left.

"Yes," I say without thanking her. I've not had time to look at the two pages.

I had called ahead to let Eric know I was not able to pick up the Cyclosporine because Dr. Anthony had not yet called Bruce, the Walgreens pharmacist, to tell him it was OK.

"That's all right," Eric says. "Just come to the pharmacy before you go. I have some free Cyclosporine to tide you over until the scrip is straightened out."

As soon as I thank Eric and hang up, Melanie, the scheduler from the Home Care agency arrives and wants to know when they can schedule Steve's visits for physical therapy, occupational therapy and nursing.

"Oh, thanks so much for coming, Melanie, it's good to meet you finally, but I don't have his schedule yet." I love the home care staff. The therapists who arrived after Steve's first discharge were all top notch.

I ask Kelly about Steve's upcoming schedule of blood draws, doctor visits and tests. She says she doesn't know and leaves the room. I slide over to the nurse's desk and take a gander at the papers Kelly had had in her hands a few minutes ago. The schedule! I flip through it to get the info Melanie needs, fold it up and put it in my jacket pocket.

Kelly returns, not saying a word. She just finishes removing Steve's bandages.

Eric stops by. I ask about the Seroquel. He says he'll make sure Walgreens has that available for Steve as well as the Cyclosporine.

I tell Steve I have to run downstairs to the hospital pharmacy and pick up the Cyclosporine Eric has left for me.

When I return, Shirley, the social worker, is waiting for me in the hallway. She tells me there's no chance of rehab, after all. I've got nothing left to say. Nothing.

We're on our own now.

As Robin Williams once said, "Joke 'em if they can't take a fuck."

Chapter Twenty-Three

So Now You Tell Me?

Tuesday, April 14, 2015
6:00 p.m.

A t last, we straggle into the apartment, warriors fresh from
the kill zone, needing some R&R. So far so good. Steve
moves with his walker in a slow deliberate fashion. Slow is good.
If he takes a tumble, I'll not be able to catch him or peel him off
the floor. I'll have to dial 911.

Fluffy remains faithful even though I've not had much time
to talk with her, other than to set out food and water and tell
her I hope she is having a nice day. She's not that much different
from a human—all she wants is loving attention, understanding,
validation, food, and pets. Not so much to ask, is it? If I had had
more time, I would have asked around about her living situation.
If no home, I'd have contacted the local Humane society to see if
we could find her a forever one.

I'm worried about Girly Girl, my favorite tabby at the colony
back in California. I call her my Guide Cat because every time I
stroll down the hill and call out for her, she comes trotting up to
me, meowing, "About time!"

She loves to walk several yards in front of me as we head down the blacktop path. It's as if she thinks the puny human behind her might get lost if she doesn't lead her to the next feeding station.

Once, just to mess with her, I started zigzagging behind her. She turned around to make sure I was following, fixed me with a green-eyed stare, and smacked my leg, as if to say, "Do not do that!" I apologized, of course, and from then on walked obediently in a straight line behind her.

I've been in touch regularly with my feeders since Steve and I left in March. I had told all of them that if anything bad happened at the colony while I was away to please not tell me since I had more than enough to fret about with Steve. One of the feeders let it slip in an email that she hadn't seen Girly Girl for several days. I had to quickly tuck that sentence into my dissociation folder. Nothing I can do until I return home.

I'm thrilled that housekeeping has come again to tidy up—counters gleaming, fresh sheets and blankets tucked in, garbage hauled away, carpet vacuumed. I'm grateful for all the help.

I haul in a box of gear from the hospital—the free Cyclosporine from Eric, the various creams Steve still needs, several unused bed pads, miscellaneous paraphernalia and the bunny Landon brought Steve for Easter. During the days of Steve's Prograf psychosis, he once asked the nurse to help him find his bunny. She, of course, thought he was hallucinating but decided to humor him by pretending to search for the missing plush rabbit. Bunny was hiding under one of Steve's pillows, surprising the nurse. Maybe he wasn't totally bonkers, after all.

I'm glad for all the supplies. I won't have to shop for much during the remainder of our time here. We're hoping to leave by the end of the month, or maybe sooner if Steve's recovery actually goes as planned. Happy thought, indeed.

"So, damn! We made it, darlin'," I say as we offload our belongings onto a dining room chair. "Can you believe we're still standing?"

It's nice to once again hug a sentient being instead of a pile of green, leafy vegetables. I don't know if I'll ever recover from that fright. But I do have the video if I ever want to relive the experience.

Recording videos throughout his ordeal has made it possible for me to create distance between me and his word salad; me and his bloody neck after the surgery; me and his eggplant arm and other scenes. I could pretend I was an observer, not an affected party. Dissociation gets an undeserved bad rap.

"Not quite yet," he says. "If it weren't for you, I wouldn't even be here." He sits down on the freshly made bed and switches on the TV. "No place like home!" The apartment has indeed become our home. A place of refuge from those who might harm him.

"That's for sure," I say and go outside to fetch our mail, returning with more cards and care packages from home. I toss them onto the bed. "Look how much people care for you, Steve. They've been rooting for your recovery this entire time."

"Yeah, that's been pretty nice." He opens up one of the boxes from his cousin to find homemade peanut brittle. Yes!

"Would you like something else to eat?" I say, hoping to get more real food into him. His Glucerna kick seems to have waned. "I've got some tasty veal parmesan I picked up at Whole Foods the other day. How about that?"

"Sounds good," he says and turns to an old movie, *Affair to Remember*. Cary Grant and Deborah Kerr. What could be better than that?

"How about some beet salad to go along with it?"

"Sure."

"I'll fix that and then get your pills ready."

It's a thrill to watch Steve feed himself. We adults have no recollection of what a big deal it was as a child to learn how to wield a spoon. We take such simple abilities for granted, and then are horrified when they disappear.

After we've eaten and Steve has had his pills, we allow as how there's nothing more to do but sleep! Beloved sleep.

"Good night, my sweet prince," I say and hug him. It's such a pleasure to have him hug me back.

"Thanks for everything," he says and smiles. "It's a new day. I can't wait to get back home, see our kitties and teach again!"

I stand in the shower for as much of forever as I can manage, slightly apologetic for my greedy consumption of the city's water supply. Our drought at home still persists. Soon enough, I'll have to resume water rationing.

I read myself to sleep, taking in Jack Reacher's latest shenanigans. That Lee Child—how does he do it?

Wednesday, April 15, 2015
7:00 a.m.

I get up much earlier than I'd like, but we're due at the transplant lab by 8:30 for another blood draw. Mustn't be tardy.

Steve it is not eager to rise and shine, but we make it to the lab on time. Steve's walking is becoming more and more steady and quick-footed. I'd hate for Nelly to scold me. And make no mistake, it would be me she scolded, not Steve.

We return to the apartment to wait for the parade of home care therapists to arrive. First the nurse, then the occupational and physical therapists. They're all amazed that Steve is doing so well, especially after his psychotic meltdown. Seems Steve has become something of a legend around the hospital for his brute strength, even post-transplant. The therapists plan to visit him twice a week for a few days and taper off as he gets stronger and stronger. I tell them we hope to leave in a couple of weeks.

Friday, April 17, 2015
9:30 a.m.

The one-month anniversary of Steve's liver transplant. Has it only been one month? Why does it feel like a year? Or a decade?

We drive to the hospital where Steve meets with a nurse's assistant to remove his abdominal staples—sixty-nine in a clear chevron pattern. I watch and video the procedure as she carefully employs a staple remover, not unlike the ones used for removing them from paper.

Steve says he feels no pain. Remarkable. He's had little pain throughout his entire ordeal. By taking videos, I have been able to keep some objective distance, as if the rancid goings on have been happening to someone other than a person I love and am forever worried about.

Steve is still very skinny, weighing only 167.5. He wants to get up to 185 or 190 before we return home. He's thrilled that he can eat whatever he wants as much as he wants with the exception of sugar and salt. Like that's gonna happen.

After we return to the apartment, the physical therapist arrives to take Steve outside for a walk around the gardens. I tag along for a while, then return inside to begin work on a rough cut of the documentary I hope to create. My videographer friend, Arnie, in California, recommended a simple video editing program, and I'm now trying, without success, to download it. I call my computer guru, Denny, and he directs me to first download all the updates available for my laptop. I do that and as if by magic I can now install the editing program. I want to complete this project before we leave. I'm afraid I might not get around to finishing it after we return to California.

I review all the video clips and select fifteen to plunk into the editing tool. The finished product, though rough, has a terrific story arc—From Normal to Psychotic to Normal again.

SCENES:

1. Steve sitting in his wheelchair in the emergency room, waiting for the nurse to take us into the patient room from which he will be moved to the operating room.

2. Steve in the ICU several hours after surgery, with his left arm the size of an eggplant, swollen and purple.

3. Steve's skeletal neck with blood oozing out of the right side.

4. Steve walking and talking on the transplant unit, getting ready for discharge.

5. Steve back in the apartment, looking like crap but able to talk and walk like a normal person.

6. Steve, the day after Prograf was doubled: can hardly walk with the walker, even with Landon at his side; cannot speak in anything other than word salad, cannot heed a one-step command.

7. Steve in full word salad mode, talking to Landon. Cannot open his mouth for food or drink and cannot swallow his anti-rejection pills.

8. Steve back at the apartment after he was switched to Cyclosporine. He's returned to his pre-Prograf days, lucid and normal in spite of having almost killed himself by yanking the hard laminate panel under the sink free from its steel bolts, and clobbering himself in the head with it.

And yet, even after using Mike Tyson force against his forehead, a normal CAT scan. Go figure.

Tuesday, April 21, 2015
8:30 a.m.

No need for labs this morning.

Home Care nurse comes at 11:30. She's impressed with Steve's recovery.

Appointment with endocrine doctor at 2:30 p.m., to discuss the risk of diabetes due to his anti-rejection drugs and the importance of a low-sugar, low-carb diet.

Appointment with Dr. Anthony at 3:20 p.m. who is also pleased with Steve's recovery. He thinks a return to California is possible in a couple of weeks or sooner. Whoo-hoo!

Return to the apartment where Steve decides to make French toast, without my help and without the benefit of his walker. At this rate, we will be flying home soon. I start to organize all our belongings in preparation for our return to California. I set up an empty box in my bedroom and start tossing in the stuff that I can't pack in my suitcase. I plan to ship it from the post office the day before we fly out.

My beloved older brother Robert and his wife Cheryl arrive from Illinois, after having driven for a few days to get here. My bro does not like to fly, a hangover from his military days, I suspect, although he never talks about it. He and Steve get along like a house afire. I've known Cheryl since second grade. They still live in our small home town, with their children nearby.

Robert and I were very close as kids. He's the childhood friend who taught me how to bowl, I, 15, he 17; who taught me how to drive a stick shift in his ancient Ford; who saved me from the prying, play-doctor eyes of the neighbor boys when I was three, he five; who put me in his little red wagon when I was four after I crashed his big tricycle on an out-of-control skid down the steep hill next to our house, breaking my arm and going into shock. He pulled me in the wagon with one hand, the tricycle in the other, all the way up the hill and walked me into our living room where Mom was having a ladies' church meeting.

I came home from the hospital, my arm in a cast, not remembering anything that happened after I crashed, except that Robert had saved me.

I've always been grateful for this kind, caring man, who grew up to be nothing like our depressed angry father. Robert even loaned me money to get away to college after our father refused to help, demanding instead that I stay home and go to secretarial school. I paid him back, with interest.

All my life my brother has been my fail-safe, the one I could count on.

Cheryl and I have been friends since we were seven when her family moved to town. We played with her sweet dog Rex at our local park. I envied her because she could do perfect cartwheels.

Although I was athletic in other ways, my feeble attempt at cartwheels always landed me on my ass. I cheered when I heard that she and my brother got together after his divorce several years ago.

Cheryl and I decide to leave the boys to solve the world's problems while we play tourist for the next few days. I feel as if I've been let out of jail, getting to bomb around the town in our little Kia Rio—window shopping, lunching, gossiping and going to the museums. I hate to say good-bye when they leave.

Sunday, April 28, 2015

Steve continues to do well, only needing his walker when going outside or to the bathroom. He pushes himself every day to get stronger and is gradually increasing the amount of food he can eat.

We see Dr. Anthony, Steve's surgeon, again for a check-up. Once again, he is happy with Steve's recovery. He wants to do a routine ultrasound of Steve's abdomen, just to see how his liver is doing. If all goes well, we can probably return home in two to three weeks, not soon enough for our taste, but Dr. A is the man whose expertise saved Steve's life, so we'll just have to chill and follow his recommendations.

Monday, May 4, 2015
8:30 a.m.

I drive Steve to the hospital for the uneventful ultrasound of his abdomen. Then home for another round of physical therapy outside on the apartment grounds. He's been discharged from occupational therapy since he is independent in all of his activities of daily living, including showering himself with the help of the shower bench I brought in several weeks ago.

I love the peace and quiet. I know that decompression won't happen overnight, that it will take a long time to recover from all the stress of the past five months. It helps that I can leave Steve in the living room with his books and television. I'm not used to all-Steve-all-the-time. Or all-anyone-all-the-time, for that matter.

I need to have undisturbed access to my mind without interruptions from one more thing and one more thing and one more damn thing. Now that I have quiet time, a memory bubbles up that I didn't have time to fully process the moment it happened.

After Steve's horrific melt-down on the transplant unit when he hit himself in the head with a board, a nurse practitioner whose name I cannot recall came over to talk to me. I was bemoaning the fact that no one had listened to me except for the two nurses who told me that Steve's crazy behavior was all because of Prograf. I withheld their names.

She told me that the surgeons wanted their patients to stay on Prograf for as long as possible after surgery to protect their livers, no matter what.

No matter what!? Her meta-message? All along, the doctors had known that Steve's problems were due to Prograf and because they wanted him to continue, they refused to tell me the truth?

That would explain why each time we took Steve to the ER, the docs avoided eye contact when they spoke to us. If only they'd told us the truth and given us an end date when Steve could safely be switched to Cyclosporine we might have gone along with their plan. We could have calmed ourselves and reassured Steve that we knew the cause of his craziness and that it would be over soon. But, no. They chose to lie and lie and lie again, leading us to think they did not know what was causing his deterioration, thus causing the man I love to nearly kill himself.

There is no forgiveness for that. And no lawsuit big enough to punish their crime, if it had come down to that.

I hope they learned their lesson.

Wednesday, May 6, 2015
10:30 a.m.

I receive a phone call from Dr. Anthony's assistant informing me that the ultrasound revealed some sort of problem in Steve's hepatic artery. He scheduled Steve for an angiogram on Thursday. Dr. Anthony wants to make certain that the problem is fixed before we return to California. The assistant wants to know if I have any questions.

I have nothing to say. Inside, I am screaming *What? No! No! No!* Thunderstruck by this berserker piece of news, I feel as though my fingers have been knocked off home row and I can no longer make out the print on the page—nothing makes sense. Nothing.

Will this liver horror never end?

I've used up everything I had to get us this far, and now I have to go back to the well? What if I have nothing left? What if I just can't do it? What if I don't want to?

A few minutes ago, I was packing for our return home, but now—

Like I've said before, if you want to make God laugh, tell her your plans.

Chapter Twenty-Four

PLEASE MAKE THIS WORK

Thursday, May 7, 2015
9:30 a.m.

I drive Steve to the hospital for a non-invasive CT angiogram. While it may be non-invasive for his physical body, for us—our hearts and spirits—it is very invasive. If anything bad happens to his hepatic artery, the liver will fail. Steve would then require another liver transplant; if one is not available in time, he will die.

A few hours later at the apartment, Dr. Anthony phones us with the results, saying the CT angiogram revealed a hair pin twist in Steve's hepatic artery, perhaps caused by the size of Steve's new liver, which is very large. This condition occurs in 3.1%-7.4% of liver transplant patients.

"What can be done about that?" I ask, holding my breath.

"I've scheduled Steve for a meeting with Dr. Bernstein tomorrow. He's a vascular surgeon and will talk to you about an angioplasty and stent."

"Uh, how dangerous is this?"

"There's always some risk, but Dr. Bernstein has done a lot of these; so there shouldn't be a problem."

"OK, then. I guess we'll see him tomorrow, then. Thanks." I hang up, dread pressing on my heart.

I explain everything to Steve. I expect him to be worried, but instead, he just shrugs and says, "Well, let's get 'er done and get out of here!"

Friday, May 8, 2015
2:30 p.m.

We meet with Dr. Bernstein, an affable, white-haired surgeon, in his office. He has reviewed Steve's records and says on Monday he plans to perform an angioplasty and install a stent in Steve's hepatic artery. He describes the procedure very matter-of-factly, says he does these all the time, not to worry.

He doesn't know it, but I'm the wrong person to tell not to worry.

We drive home in silence. We had thought of playing tourist on Saturday to check out the city, maybe even eat at a restaurant, anything but raw seafood or a buffet. Steve has been told in no uncertain terms that he cannot eat sushi or any raw fish, nor should he frequent a salad bar. His immune system is now compromised and any bacteria or virus could bring him down.

Steve says, "I think we should stick close to home this weekend, don't you?"

"I agree," I say, relieved. If anything should happen over the weekend, I can get Steve to the hospital in fifteen minutes. Instead of winging it to California in a week as we had hoped, I will be in the waiting room, hoping Dr. Bernstein can fix Steve's twisty artery.

We spend our time watching TV, walking around the gardens, admiring the tulips and daffodils and other assorted flowering plants, petting Fluffy, and not talking about Monday. I email family and friends about this new development.

Monday, May 11, 2015
8:00 a.m.

We meet with Dr. Bernstein prior to the procedure. He explains that Steve will be given a light sedative, that he will insert a catheter into one of Steve's femoral arteries, snake it up to the hair pin turn and install the stent. Easy peasy. He didn't actually say "easy peasy;" that's just my magical thinking at work.

Unable to concentrate on a magazine, I clutch my cell phone and pace around the waiting room, as if constant motion will stave off the bad juju. Dr. Bernstein has said the procedure would take about an hour.

After two hours, Dr. Bernstein finally returns to the waiting room to tell me that he was unable to seat the stent. Steve's arteries are too twisty and he couldn't get around them.

"Uh, that can't be good. Now what?" I run my fingers through my hair, barely breathing.

Not again.

"Dr. Anthony will talk with you about that," he says, eager to leave and get onto his next case.

"Oh. Is Steve OK?"

"Yes, he's fine. He'll be ready to leave in about forty-five minutes."

After Steve is released, I drive us slowly back to the apartment.

"Well, that's a kick in the head, right?" I say.

"It is what it is," Steve says.

We return to the apartment and wait to hear from Dr. Anthony. I shove aside the box I had been packing in my bedroom. Who knows when we will be able to leave? California and our cats will have to wait. Sugar and Billy continue to do well, but I know they miss us.

"It's too bad that Dr. Bernstein couldn't get your artery fixed," I say when I return to the living room. I don't tell Steve how worried I am, but I want to suss out his level of anxiety.

"I'm sure Dr. Anthony will think of something. I know this is serious but I'm not overly worried about it."

Steve's sanguine response both comforts and irritates me.

Tuesday, May 12, 2015

Unbeknownst to us, an emergency meeting of the seven transplant surgeons was called to discuss treatment options. I was told later that they actually took a vote. A vote?!! Better than throwing dice, I guess, or the I Ching.

The result was as follows: One surgeon voted to do nothing except prescribe Plavix, a blood thinner (now acceptable because Steve's platelets had climbed to 100,000) and send him home where, if a problem developed, he could be taken care of by the transplant team at the University of California San Francisco where he'd been on the waiting list. I'm sure they would have loved that.

Another surgeon voted to perform major surgery on the hepatic artery itself, but that was deemed too risky because they'd not done many of those procedures at this hospital. Still another suggested they consult with an interventional radiologist who had extensive experience with twisty veins and ask him to take a stab at stenting Steve's hepatic artery.

The last option won. Dr. Anthony, determined to make sure Steve's artery was fixed before they released him to California, contacted Dr. Carr, described to us as a genius interventional radiologist who could fix almost anything. Steve was scheduled for the procedure on Thursday.

Thursday, May 14, 2015
3:30 a.m.

I wake up at 3:30 a.m. to prepare us for Steve's procedure. I wolf down a quick breakfast, grab some snacks and a bottle of green tea and stuff them, along with my back pillow, into my tote. This could be a very long day. I ready Steve's pills. He was given the OK to take them with a few sips of water before his appointment.

"Rise and shine, Honey, this is your big day," I say as if we're off to the county fair where Steve will show off his prize-winning White Rock chickens. He rolls out of bed and walks himself to the bathroom, sans walker. His strength is returning more and more each day.

He dresses himself with alacrity, but still needs help with his pressure socks. Those are a bitch to don alone.

"What do you think about taking your walker, just in case? You might need it after the procedure."

"Sure." He navigates with it on the way out to the car, then folds it up and sets it in the trunk. I'm proud of him for carrying through with all his exercises. His diligence is paying off. It will be much easier to travel with him, now that his belly is not so huge and his balance is better. I picture the redwood trees outside our patio and can feel the California breeze on my face. That's where I want us to be, not here where the bad things happen.

My heart skips a few beats as I drive, thinking about the Google search I had conducted. Hairpin turns of the hepatic artery are tricky business, and fixing them associates with high morbidity. I do not share this info with Steve.

We meet with Dr. Carr, a forty-something doctor with intelligent brown eyes whose reputation for excellence precedes him. He displays the confident mien you want in someone who holds the life or death of your loved one in his hands.

He explains the procedure, the light sedative and the snaking of the catheter through one of Steve's arteries, to be chosen at the time he and his team assess Steve. I give Steve a buss on the cheek.

"See ya." He smiles and waves.

"Don't worry," Dr. Carr says, "we'll take good care of him." I nod and leave.

I scuff over to the cavernous waiting room where it all started on March 17, nearly two long, tortured months ago, only this time it's not 1:30 a.m., and my body is not splayed over the three hard burgundy ottomans.

The room is three-quarters filled with family members, some with children, waiting for word that their loved one has weathered their surgery and is going to be fine.

Worry drenches the room, leaking all over their nonchalance.

I don't know why, but I'm more worried about this procedure than I was about the transplant. I was naïve and didn't know then what I know now about how things can go wrong.

One surgeon, Dr. Bernstein, has already failed to fix Steve's tricky artery.

How do we know that Dr. Carr will succeed?

I've located a table and chair as far away from the madding crowd as possible. Waiting, wound tight, convinced that if I let go and relax, the shit will hit the fan and it will be my fault. The only thing keeping Steve alive is my vigilance—a foolhardy belief, I know, but I've never imagined that any omnipotent, omniscient God would drop all his plans to attend to me or to Steve and I've no other strategy to cling to.

Everyone in the waiting room is on a razor's edge but pretending to be otherwise, playing with their children as if this were just another play date; the children scrambling, scrapping with each other, acting out their parents' unspoken fears. The parents, distracted, fail to shush their children's screeching. I want to scream, "Shut up, shut up, you're killing me!" I need to concentrate, as though keeping myself wound up will help Steve. I should know better, but I'm having an amygdala highjack and that's the best I can do.

I've gone feral again, my senses heightened and on the prowl: the blaze of clashing colors from their clothing; the crunch of nails being bitten; every hiccup of the air conditioner; kids crawling on the scruffy floor, their shoes squeaking; brows knitting; the reception desk phone ringing; the murmur of voices low on cell phones; the sniffling and snuffling; wild bursts of laughter fueled by the wild bursts of fear in their hearts; snoring; teeming masses huddled; limbs splashing over the arms of the chairs. Some have been here for hours, possibly overnight, waiting, waiting, hoping, praying; the smell of burgers and fries, brought in to sustain.

I open a book, a prop to keep my eyes entertained while the brain is occupied elsewhere—in the operating room, overseeing the surgery, praying, yet not praying, visualizing success. What's taking so long?

Ninety minutes later, Dr. Carr walks slowly toward me from the surgical suite. I laser in on his face, his body language—is his stride halting as though the last thing he wants to do is talk to me? Are his shoulders hunched forward and down? Have the creases of his nasolabial folds deepened? Does he have a squint to his eyes? I scour him for any signs of defeat. Holding my breath, I massage my forehead with one hand as I stand up and place the other on the table to steady myself.

"Mrs. West?" he says and smiles, reaching for my hand, which I gladly turn over to him. "I want to update you on our progress so that you won't worry." I nod stupidly.

"We've run into a few snags," he says.

Snags? Snags? We don't like snags.

"The first femoral artery we chose to insert the catheter and stent into didn't allow for us to get close enough to the hepatic artery. We've got a few other moves to make. I've got a great team—another interventional radiologist and a neurosurgeon—working on your husband, and I'm confident we will succeed."

He's so kind, I tear up; all I can do is bobble my head and eke out a "Thank you." He actually seems to care, not just about Steve, but about how I might be feeling as I wait. I could kiss him for that. I believe him when he says he is confident he will succeed.

"I just wanted you to know that this will take longer than we expected, and I didn't want you to worry." How can he be so calm when he has someone's life in his hands?

"Oh, that's very kind of you. I appreciate that," I say in a monotone, not much energy available for prosody today.

Is he lying to me? Is Steve already dead? Should I make plans for that? But, no, my gut signals that Dr. Carr is telling the truth. And I have to believe that, at least for now. What choice do I have?

But what if we've come this far, only to lose Steve at the last minute because of some stupid blockage? What if our suffering has all been for naught—the pain, terror, anxiety, anger—and find in the end that there's nothing more I can do? That would kill me.

I recall an old friend who was fond of saying, "Time to leave the party; the ice cream's turned to shit." I never asked him what he meant exactly, but I assume it means, "Don't overstay your welcome." Have we overstayed our welcome at this hospital?

I know it sounds stupid, but everything seems stupid right now. My mind goes wild, rewinding the events to date: the hash they made of their case management system, right out of the chute. More like their case mangled system: the snafus during the evaluation week that led us to the ER when all Steve needed was Lactulose to stem the encephalopathy and confusion. It's not as though I hadn't alerted the social worker and the gastroenterologist about this on the very first day of our evaluation.

But because neither one of them took action to send Steve for a simple blood test and then treat him with Lactulose, I had to make several frantic calls to the social worker in the afternoon about Steve's increasing confusion. Because my calls were ignored, we ended up in the ER where the surgical resident came mighty close to administering a potentially fatal dose of heparin. Then management blamed me for not using the word "urgent" in my phone calls, the recordings of which later mysteriously disappeared. The recordings would have corroborated my story that I had indeed said the word urgent. Then, after Steve's transplant, the doubling up of Prograf and the doctors' refusal to tell me what was going on, leaving Landon and me to deal with Steve's psychosis during which he almost killed himself.

Where was the fail-safe when we needed it most?

I cannot will Steve to stay alive, no matter the strength of my intention, and I fear it is naive to trust the surgeons; so where does that leave me? Hope? Hope is stupid. Hope is bullshit. Hope is only worthwhile if it fuels action. I might be a tad bitter.

I look around at the other family members in the waiting room and want to scream: Do you know what's happening right now to your husband, wife, sister, brother, child? Did you arm yourself with information before the surgery? Do you know exactly what's happening—the risks and the benefits? The options other than surgery? Did you research the best places and surgeons to do this surgery? Do you know what medications he or she is taking? Are you aware of their potential side effects? Do you know her or his medical history, inside and out? Are you prepared to confront their doctors if something seems not right, or do you just "trust" them and hope for the best?

Which of your loved ones is going to be added to the long list of patients who will die this year because of a preventable medical error? Which one of you will spring into action to make sure that doesn't happen? Odds are that at least one won't make it out of surgery today because someone has screwed up.

I hope it won't be Steve.

Chapter Twenty-Five

AT LAST: HOME TO CALIFORNIA

Thursday, May 14, 2015
3:00 p.m.

Vigilance is exhausting; I'm running out of adrenaline and need to go to bed. For the past three hours, I've been listening to the names of the other family members as they are announced on the public address system. One by one they quickly gather up their belongings and scurry toward the entrance to the surgical suite and disappear inside. Since they do not return to the waiting room by the same door, I assume there is another exit. Wouldn't do for the rest of us to be exposed to screaming, bawling, seething, heartbroken families. Maybe this is everyone's lucky day and they all exit happily.

I notice Dr. Carr walking swiftly toward me from the surgical suite, and before I can concoct any scary stories, he says, "It's done. He's fine." The four finest words in the English language. *It's done. He's fine.* Now I can cry.

"Oh, my God." My lips tremble. "You have no idea how worried I've been," I leap up and hug him. "There are not enough words to thank you for saving my sweetheart."

"You're welcome," he says and pulls away slowly from the lady with the tears. "I'm glad it turned out well. We're going to keep Mr. West overnight, just to make sure everything is OK."

"When can I see him?" I strap on my fanny pack, toss my book, my uneaten sandwich, and back pillow into my tote bag.

"Follow me." He turns around and strides off. I'm just one of many people Dr. Carr will talk to that day. I don't know how he does it. `

He leads me to the recovery section of the surgical suite where, under the bright fluorescent lights, Steve is sitting up, sipping some water, attended to by a nice young nurse named Walter. Steve nods toward Dr. Carr and says, "This man is every bit the genius they said he was. I feel fine." Steve looks much better than he should—with his pretty wavy gray hair and his skin returning to its previous healthy glow, given all he's been through. I suspect his own dissociation machine has been working overtime.

"Well," Dr. Carr says and laughs, "you certainly put us through our paces with those twisty veins of yours, Mr. West. We're glad we succeeded."

"When can I go home?"

"We need to keep you just for tonight, and then wait a few days to see how your repeat ultrasounds turn out. We want to make sure everything is stable before we can discharge you, but I imagine it will be soon."

"Yay!" I say. "We're ready, right Sweetheart?" and thrust my fist in the air.

"Hell yeah," he says, grinning, "More than ready."

"Well, I'll leave you to it, then," Dr. Carr says. "We'll be in touch about your ultrasound schedule." And, with that, he slips out the door, on the way to save another lucky person. All in a day's work.

Monday, May 18, 2015

The following days are shockingly free of horror. Only one slight hiccup four days after Dr. Carr successfully performed the angioplasty and installed the stent. Steve's new ultrasound shows improved blood flow, but not enough to satisfy him or Dr. Anthony, Steve's transplant surgeon.

Wednesday, May 20, 2015

Steve undergoes a repeat ultrasound. Afterward, Nelly calls to say that the blood flow is getting better. I ask her about a discharge date for Steve and how much longer he would need to take the blood thinner Plavix. Grumpy as ever, she growls that she will contact Dr. Carr and get back to us. Hell might freeze over.

In the meantime, we begin to think of ourselves as normal people, just here on a vacay, dontcha know. It's true that anyone could tell that Steve is still severely underweight, what with his sunken cheeks and his skinny arms and legs, and that for us "normal" is aspirational, but we believe it to be on its way.

I'm astounded that we survived the past five months. What I need most now is no more drama so I can process everything that's happened—a fierce transformation thrust upon me, piercing through layers of midwestern politeness and obedience, scores of childhood interactions that solidified in us girls and women the belief that no one would like us if we kicked up a fuss.

People liking us was the be all and end all of our existence.

Well, that's now dead and buried.

For our first outings in months, we dine at a top-rated restaurant one evening and on another evening at a Mexican restaurant our neighbors had recommended. Even though he remains skinny, the Steve I've known and loved for sixteen years has re-emerged despite the ongoing fatigue. His linguistic brain has returned; word salad has packed up its tongs and bowl and left the dining room.

We discuss the new book we were working on together before the transplant—*The Vibrant English Verb: Mastering Meaning and Usage.* Steve's special gift for explaining complicated verb forms comes alive in his classes of TESOL students so that they can not only understand them, but can teach real world usage to non-native English Learners. What they need now is a textbook to match. I've designed the cover and am editing Steve's sometimes convoluted prose. Then, when all is done, Mr. Amazon and I will see that it gets uploaded properly.

It's just a matter of time before we hear the words "You are free to go." I rush around, doing laundry, packing the box we will be sending to California, schlepping it to the post office and donating the shower bench and walker to a non-profit organization providing services for the disabled. I clean the refrigerator, give away food and Steve's huge pre transplant clothes to our neighbor whose husband is a husky man. I write a thank you note to the housekeeping staff who have lightened our load.

I walk to the Oasis restaurant, just as I did our first night in this new city, for some veggie wraps. Seems like decades ago.

Steve brightens the day for family and friends with his phone calls. They are very surprised and happy to hear from him, eager to see us in the flesh once again.

After we return home to California, Steve plans to write and send a letter to the donor family, via the hospital staff, who will forward it on to them. Even though we might never receive a response, we want them to know of our profound gratitude for their gift of life, and that their father/brother/son/uncle/cousin lives on in a grateful man named Steve.

Friday, May 22, 2015
1:00 p.m.

We finally get the call—Steve is free to go. Oh my God! It's really happening; we are going home. Before we do, we head to the transplant office to sign some papers. We also stop by the office of Dr. Anthony, who happens to be in, and we thank him over and over again for saving Steve's life. He stands up and opens his arms for our hugs.

"This day is a gift for me, too," he says. "This is why I do what I do."

"Good-bye," we say in unison.

Sunday, May 24, 2015
12:00 p.m.

Finally! We collect our bags, take them to the Kia Rio for our last ride. Just as we are about to pull away, we notice Fluffy sitting next to the curb, staring at us. This is the first and only time she's followed us to the parking lot.

Does she know this is the last time she will see us? I turn off the ignition, step out of the car to pet her and thank her for being there for us every day when we returned to the apartment. I tear up when I tell her good-bye. She's been our faithful friend for all these months, such a love. If I could have scooped her up and taken her with us, I would have.

She'd like California.

4:00 p.m.

We are finally cleared for take-off, in every sense of the word, seated aboard United Airlines, buckled up, bags stowed, holding hands and smiling. No one on this plane knows what a gift Steve is bringing home with him—a new liver, a new life.

No one knows what hell we had to endure to get it and to keep it.

I wish for all of them long healthy lives, free of medical catastrophe.

END NOTES FOR MAIN TEXT

1. Chronic Stress Puts Your Health at Risk. August 1, 2023. https://www.mayoclinic.org/healthy-lifestyle/stress-management/in-depth/stress/art-20046037

2. The Sociology of Gaslighting. *American Sociological Review*, 2019, Vol.84(5) 851-875 https://www.asanet.org/wp-content/uploads/attach/journals/oct19asrfeature.pdf

3. *The Assault on Truth: Freud's Suppression of the Seduction Theory by Jeffrey Moussaieff* Masson, 1985, Penguin Books

4. A Comparison of Tacrolimus (FK506) and Cyclosporine for Immunosuppression in Liver Transplantation. N. England Journal of Medicine 1994, https://pubmed.ncbi.nlm.nih.gov/7523946/

5. Akinetic Mutism Induced by Tacrolimus (Prograf) https://pubmed.ncbi.nlm.niih.gov/19820432, Sep-Oct, 2009

6. Mutism and Persistent Dysarthria due to Tacrolimus-based Immunosupprssion Following Allogenic Liver Transplantation. https://pubmed.ncbi.nlm.nih.gov/20535006/

7. Manic-Like Psychosis Associated with Elevated Tacrolimus (Prograf) Concentrations 17 years After Kidney Transplant. https://www.hindawi.com/journals/crips/2013/926395/

8. Akinetic Mutism—A Review of the Literature. https://pubmed.ncbi.nlm.nih.gov/7705740/2007

9. https://gutivate.com/blog/is-my-doctor-gaslighting-me#:~:text=Medical%20gaslighting%20refers%20to%20the,perception%20of%20their%20health%20condition.

10. https://www.verywellhealth.com/signs-of-gaslighting-5219024#:~:text=It%20is%20often%20present%20in,trivializing%2C%20with%20holding%2C%20or%20diverting.

11. https://www.choosingtherapy.com/medical-gaslighting/

PART 2

ADDENDUM

In this section I share insights and knowledge that I've acquired since we returned home with Steve's new liver. I wish I had been armed with this information before Steve's transplant. The material presented is not meant to be exhaustive, but rather intended to highlight important healthcare issues. I don't claim to have solutions to all these problems, but I do believe that the first step toward change is to acknowledge and understand their existence.

For a more in-depth understanding, please consult the list of Resources I've included at the end.

I. Medical Errors

In 2016, Johns Hopkins University reported that 251,000 people died every year from preventable medical errors.[1] (please see End Notes) Their data included medical errors of all types, including the medical errors to which Steve was subjected.

In 2023, researchers from Johns Hopkins and Harvard came to an even more startling conclusion: 371,000 patients die every year from medical errors and 424,000 are permanently disabled.[2] Their data included only diagnostic errors, not surgical errors or medication errors.

The top fifteen conditions associated with the errors investigated in their study were: stroke, myocardial infarction, venous thromboembolism, aortic aneurysm, arterial thrombosis, sepsis, meningitis, encephalitis, spinal abscess, pneumonia, endocarditis, lung cancer, breast cancer, colorectal cancer, prostate cancer and melanoma.

In other words, these are the illnesses for which doctors may fail to diagnose your symptoms correctly, and you or a loved one may suffer injury or death as a result.

Five of these conditions accounted for nearly 40% of all cases of death and permanent disability: stroke, sepsis, pneumonia, lung cancer, and pulmonary embolism.

Strokes were missed 18% of the time, leading to 94,000 deaths and disabilities.

"We were not surprised by the large number of serious harms from diagnostic error, but we were surprised to find that half of them are attributable to just 15 diseases and nearly 40 percent are attributable to just five," says lead study author David Newman-Toker, MD, PhD, director of the Center for Diagnostic Excellence at Johns Hopkins Medicine in Baltimore, July, 2023.[3]

The number of medical errors revealed in both studies is staggering. The number of patients and family members who suffer as a result is even more staggering.

II. Medication Errors

Medication errors are another potential source of death and disability. According to a report in the *New York Post,* September 4, 2023, up to 9,000 patients die every year in the U.S. as a result of a prescription medication error.[4]

"That figure doesn't (even) include the hundreds of thousands of patients who suffer adverse effects from taking the wrong medication or taking meds in the wrong way."

The Los Angeles Times reported on September 23, 2023 that pharmacies in California make an estimated 5 million errors every year![5]

Ellen Gabler, investigative reporter for *The New York Times,* January 31, 2020, interviewed pharmacists from all over the country.[6] According to her reporting, "They struggle to fill prescriptions, give flu shots, tend the drive-through, answer phones, work the register, counsel patients and call doctor and insurance companies, they said—all the while racing to meet corporate performance metrics that they characterize as unreasonable and unsafe in an industry squeezed to do more with less."

One pharmacist in Texas went so far as to send an anonymous letter to the Texas State Board of Pharmacy, saying, "I am a danger to the public working for CVS."

NBC reported that pharmacists employed by the large chains, CVS, Walgreens and Rite Aid staged a three-day walkout in early November, 2023.[7]

Since pharmacists are not unionized, they were putting their jobs on the line on behalf of patient safety by asking, not for more pay but for more help. One worker complained that often she could not even take a bathroom break.

The report continues on to point out that The American Pharmacists Association and National Alliance of State Pharmacy Associations conducted a survey in 2021 which revealed the following: 74% of 4,482 pharmacy workers polled said they didn't have enough time to safely perform nonclinical work and 75% said there were not enough other staff, like techs and nurses, to safely perform clinical work.

All of this is happening at a time when the three biggest drugstore chains have all begun closing stores. CVS is planning to close 900 locations in three years. Walgreens said in June of 2023 that it would close 150 U.S. locations. Rite Aid is also closing at least 154 stores and maybe more since it's going through Chapter 11 bankruptcy reorganization.

III. Burnout and Moral Injury

When health care providers, i.e. doctors, nurses, pharmacists and others are forced to do too much with too little, patient harm can ensue. You might think that the solution would be obvious: hire more employees.

You'd be morally right, of course, but economically wrong. More hours for workers = less profit for owners.

Dr. Eric Reinhart, a physician at Northwestern University, published a heartfelt essay in *The New York Times*, February 5, 2023: "Doctors Aren't Burned Out From Overwork. We're Demoralized by Our Health System." [8]

In it, he says, "The United States is the only high-income nation that doesn't provide universal health care to its citizens. Instead, it maintains a lucrative system of for-profit medicine."

He points out that the pressure to produce more and more revenue for these systems has led to 117,000 physicians leaving the field in 2021. At the same time, fewer than 40,000 have joined the field.

As far back as July, 2018, a study led by Stanford University researchers claimed that "The epidemic of physician burnout may be the source of even more medical errors than unsafe medical workplace conditions.[9]

According to the Health Resources and Services Administration, May 4, 2024, the U.S. needs more than 17,477 additional primary care practitioners, 12,834 dental health practitioners, and 8,364 mental health practitioners.[10]

The Association of American Medical Colleges has found that the United States could experience a shortfall of between 37,800 and 124,000 physicians by 2034 for both primary and specialty care, Mary 4, 2024.[11]

Wendy Dean, M.D., a psychiatrist, elaborates on the concept of "moral injury" in her groundbreaking book of 2023, *If I Betray These Words: Moral Injury in Medicine and Why It's So Hard for Clinicians to Put Patients Frst.*[12]

The idea for her book came about soon after she read an article about a physician suicide and began asking physicians how they felt about their jobs. She heard the same story over and over: they were being asked to pay more attention to their productivity than to their patients. They felt burned out from a health care system that made it difficult for them to care for their patients.

Although the term "moral injury" originated in the military, Dr. Dean felt it applied equally well to overburdened healthcare workers.

According to the website, "Open Arms Veterans and Family Counseling," moral injury refers to the psychological, social and spiritual impact of events involving betrayal or transgression of one's own deeply held moral beliefs and values occurring in high stakes situations.[13]

In other words, when soldiers or healthcare workers are forced to perform in settings that force them to violate their personal sense of morality and their professional ethics, the result for these individuals is overwhelming stress.

An article in the *New York Times*, June 15, 2023, "The Corporatization of Health Care has Changed the Practice of Medicine, Causing Many Physicians to Feel Alienated From Their Work," examines the problem in detail and quotes Dr. Dean and her co-author Simon G. Talbot: "Doctors on the front lines of America's profit-driven health care system are also susceptible to such wounds . . . as the demands of administrators, hospital executives and insurers forced them to stray from the ethical principles that were supposed to govern their profession. The pull of these forces has left many doctors anguished and distraught, caught between the Hippocratic oath and the realities of making a profit from people at their sickest and most vulnerable."[14]

IV. THE ROLE OF PRIVATE EQUITY IN HEALTH CARE

I 've been vaguely aware of the term "Private Equity" for years, most often in connection with the bankruptcies of the companies that PE companies had taken over, i.e. Toys "R" Us and others.

I had no idea these billionaire-owned companies were involved in health care until Gretchen Morgenson, author of *These are the Plunderers: How Private Equity Runs and Wrecks America*, was interviewed by Terri Gross on her program *Fresh Air*, April 26, 2023.[15]

I learned from the interview and from reading Ms. Morgenson's book how Private Equity firms buy out privately held companies, load them up with debt by using a variety of sophisticated maneuvers, then lay off employees—who lose their 401ks in the process—and cut additional costs in order to fatten their already-bloated bottom lines. After sucking the companies dry, the companies are often forced to file for bankruptcy, at no cost to the Private Equity firm.

Thousands of people have lost and will continue to lose their jobs because of the shenanigans of Private Equity. For example,

Private Equity backed retailers shed half a million jobs over the past two decades, by shuttering 18,000 stores and eliminating nearly 542,000 jobs. (October 19, 2021) [16]

All perfectly legal. All harmful to our economy, our workers, and in the case of health care, physicians, nurses and their patients, pharmacists and their customers—a danger to the public.

Tim Wu, a law professor at Columbia, in April of 2020 published an article in the *New York Times* about how "A Corporate Merger Cost America Ventilators."[17]

Who can forget the deadly onslaught of Covid in 2020-2021? And the dearth of ventilators? And bodies stacked up in refrigerated trucks outside hospitals?

Didn't have to happen.

Mr. Wu, an attorney, reported that in 2012 the FTC allowed the merger of two companies: Newport Medical Instruments, a "small developer of cheap, portable ventilators and Covidien, a much larger American Company headquartered in Ireland for tax purposes, which made larger and more expensive ventilators."

Mr. Wu says, "We now know that approving that merger without conditions had severe costs. It would cripple what had been a prescient federal program, begun in 2007, to build an emergency stockpile of up to 40,000 portable ventilators with the eventual help of Newport Medical Instruments." Covidien terminated that federal contract, apparently in large part because it was insufficiently profitable. The company didn't want cheap portable ventilators competing with their larger, more expensive models.

"The cancellation set back the federal ventilator program by at least seven years. In fact, 13 years later, in the midst of the coronavirus crisis and despite a new contract with another company, not a single ventilator has been delivered (as of 2020)."

This is what happens when government agencies do not have strong enough enforcement mechanisms in place to protect consumer interests.

How many more lives could have been saved if the Covidien company had been mandated to continue the contract so that we would have had ventilators in sufficient numbers for everyone who needed them?

For readers interested in a lengthy and detailed account of the ventilator fiasco, please see the *New York Times*, March, 2020 article: "*The U.S. Tried to Build a New Fleet of Ventilators. The Mission Failed.*"[18]

The next time you hear representatives from Big Business and/or some politicians push for "deregulation" as the solution to any and all our economic woes, think of the thousands of patients who died for lack of a ventilator.

V. Inequities in Health Care

As stressful as Steve's hospitalization was, we were grateful we had excellent health insurance which gave Steve a chance at a new life with a new liver.

Not everyone in America is so fortunate. As far we could tell, there were no Black patients on the transplant unit during our stay. From my research into medical errors, I have become aware of the extent to which Black patients are discriminated against. How can we say that the U.S. healthcare system is the best when many Americans are not only left out of care, but injured or killed when they seek it?

According to the Assistant Secretary for Planning and Evaluation of Health Policy in February, 2022, "White Americans were more likely to have private insurance coverage (73 percent) compared to Black Americans (55 percent), while Black Americans were more likely to have public insurance coverage (30 vs. 18 percent) or be uninsured (15 vs. 9 percent)."[19]

"Hispanics have the highest uninsured rates of any racial or ethnic group within the United States. In 2020, the Census Bureau reported that 49.9 percent of Hispanics had private insurance coverage, as compared to 73.9 percent for non-Hispanic whites."[20]

As a country, we are clearly not doing enough to take care of all our citizens.

Without health insurance, people often forgo preventive care, or any care at all, except perhaps at the emergency room.

As a result, medical expenses are most often the reason Americans file for bankruptcy.

A new study, February 1, 2019, from academic researchers found that 66.5 percent of all bankruptcies were tied to medical issues—either because of high costs for care or time out of work. An estimated 530,000 families turn to bankruptcy each year because of medical issues and bills.[21]

VI. RACIAL BIAS IN MEDICAL CARE AND IN AI CHATBOTS

When it comes to medical treatment, not all Americans are treated equally. Racial disparities are glaring and unforgivable.

A study entitled, "Racial Bias in Pain Assessment and Treatment Recommendations, and False Beliefs About Biological Differences Between Blacks and Whites" was reported in the "Proceedings of the National Academy of Sciences of the U.S, April 4, 2016.[22] The study was designed to examine those beliefs associated with racial bias in pain management, which are critical to the understanding and resolving of racial disparities in medical care.

The research revealed that a substantial number of white laypeople, medical students and medical residents held false beliefs about biological differences between Blacks and Whites. It further demonstrated that these beliefs resulted in racial bias when patients were treated adequately (or not) for pain.

Here's the list of the false beliefs as presented in the study about biological differences between Blacks and Whites which can influence a doctor's assessment and treatment plan for Blacks:

1. On average, Blacks age more slowly than Whites.

2. Black people's nerve endings are less sensitive than White people's nerve endings.

3. Black people's blood coagulates more quickly and because of that, Blacks have a lower rate of hemophilia than Whites.

4. Whites, on average, have larger brains than Blacks.

5. Whites have a better sense of hearing compared to Blacks.

6. Black people's skin has more collagen (i.e. it's thicker) than White people's skin.

7. Blacks have a more sensitive sense of smell than Whites; they can differentiate odors and detect faint smells better than Whites.

8. Whites have more efficient respiratory systems than Blacks.

9. Blacks are better at detecting movement than Whites.

10. Blacks have stronger immune systems than Whites and are less likely to contract colds.

Human beings, however, are not the only ones spreading misinformation.

Racial bias also exists in AI Chatbots.

The Stanford School of Medicine conducted tests on Open AI's Chat GP, Google's Bard and three other chat bots to find out whether or not they were capable of providing medical information free of bias. Their findings were reported in *Chief Heathcare Executive*, October 25, 2023.[23]

Researchers asked nine questions on five different occasions, generating 45 answers for each large language model. All of them perpetuated race-based information, including misinformation relating to kidney function, lung capacity, muscle mass, skin thickness and pain threshold.

The researchers concluded by issuing a warning for practitioners to steer clear of relying on AI bots for medical information.

VII. BLACK WOMEN AND MATERNAL DEATHS

An article was published in *ProPublica*, December 7, 2017, entitled "Nothing Protects Black Women From Dying in Pregnancy and Childbirth."[24]

Directly under the title is the following tagline: "Not education. Not income. Not even being an expert on racial disparities in health care." This latter phrase refers to Shalon Irving, 36, MA, PhD, Lieutenant Commander in the uniformed ranks of the U.S. Public Health Service and a scientist at the CDC. She specialized in the study of racial disparities in health care. None of that protected her, a Black woman, from dying a few days after delivering her first child due to complications of high blood pressure, which had not been adequately treated after delivery.

"According to the CDC, black mothers in the U.S. die at three to four times the rate of white mothers, one of the widest of all racial disparities in women's health. Put another way, a black woman is 22 percent more likely to die from heart disease than a white woman, 71 percent more likely to perish from cervical cancer, but 243 percent more likely to die from pregnancy-or childbirth-related causes. In a national study of five medical complications that are common causes of maternal death and injury, black women were two to three times more likely to die than white women who had the same condition."

Limited diversity in the medical profession may contribute to black mothers' sense of anxiety and alienation. Blacks make up of doctors, though 11 percent of OB-GYNs 3 percent of and less than 2 percent of National Institutes of Health-funded principal investigators.

Johns Hopkins published a paper on May 12, 2023, "How Can We Solve the Black Maternal Health Crisis?"[25]

In it they noted that "Black women are two to three times more likely to die from pregnancy-related complications than white women, with most of the maternal deaths being. This heightened risk spans all income and education levels. According to the study from the the wealthiest Black woman in California is at a higher risk of maternal mortality than the least wealthy white woman."

The report goes on to say, "Amid a national reckoning with the systemic racism underpinning American society and health care, advocates are pushing forward solutions from multiple angles, including reforming policy, health systems and medical education, and bolstering community-based organizations that advocate for better care and resources for Black moms."

The report provides links to many organizations that are working on this national nightmare.

What the report failed to mention, however, is that "Homicide is the leading cause of death among pregnant women and women who are six weeks postpartum. Indeed, homicide exceeds other leading causes of maternal mortality by more than twofold. . . .

Pregnant Black women are eight times more likely to be killed by their intimate partner than non-pregnant Black women."[26]

VIII. RACIAL BIAS TRAINING, MANDATED BUT STALLED IN CALIFORNIA

O n October 7, 2019 Governor Gavin Newsom of California approved and signed into law SB-464. the "California Dignity in Pregnancy and Childbirth Act."

This law was designed to root out and correct whatever racial bias exists in an institution that prevents Black women and their infants from receiving the excellent health care they require and deserve.

I've included a copy of the complete law in the "Appendix" because it demonstrates what governments can and should do when enough citizens put pressure on lawmakers to do the right thing. This law could serve as a model for other states.

So, four years after its passage, how is this law working in California?

Not as well as you might think or hope.

"California Hospitals Ignored Bias Training Despite High Black Maternal Death Rate (December 7, 2017)"[27]

According to the above report from *CalMatters,* the results of which were discussed on KQED-FM in San Francisco, October 30, 2023, "no hospitals were in compliance when the department began its investigation in 2021, and not a single employee had completed training."

"By October, 2023, only 17% of hospitals were in compliance, according to an investigation published by the state Department of Justice."

California Attorney General Rob Bonta was not pleased. At a press conference he said, "The training matters because of the state's persistently high death rates among Black mothers."

Bonta continued, "Investigations into the cause of all pregnancy-related deaths by the California Department of Public Health determined that more than half are preventable."

"We need to listen to this data. It's screaming at us to do something, "Bonta said. "Listen to these women and make substantial change before another patient is hurt or worse."

Even with a state law in place that details all the changes hospitals are required to make in order to reduce black maternal and infant deaths, the changes are not being implemented.

Additional Must Reads on this topic:

1. *Under the Skin: The Hidden Toll of Racism on American Lives and on the Health of Our Nation* by Linda Villarosa, Doubleday, 2022.

2. *Medical Apartheid: The Dark History of Medical Experimentation on Black Americans from Colonial Times to the Present* by Harriet Washington, Penguin Random House, 2008

Check out the link to the chilling video about this book by clicking on a link embedded in the article in ProPublica,

December 7, 2017 entitled "Nothing Protects Black Women From Dying in Pregnancy and Childbirth:

https://www.propublica.org/article/nothing-protects-black-women-from-dying-in-pregnancy-and-childbirth.

IX. Recommendations for Keeping a Loved One Safe in the Hospital

Disclaimer

The following information and recommendations are presented for educational purposes only. As always, your medical provider is the professional to whom you must turn for answers about your medical questions or problems.

Steve and I had to leap over many medical hurdles to save his life. There's no doubt that if I hadn't had medical experience from working in health care administration, case management and psychotherapy, I would have been in the same position as you might be in right now—trusting medical professionals to do the right thing, not knowing how to make that happen and being horrified if that trust breaks down.

I believe that people who become physicians or nurses do so because they truly want to help others. I doubt that anyone enters these difficult professions in order to do harm.

However, harm is done every day to unsuspecting patients due to any number of factors. In the most significant way, you are your loved one's fail safe.

I have simplified the following recommendations by presenting them as if you were the caretaker and were in charge of your loved one's care. But everything I highlight here pertains to you as well. The list is not meant to be exhaustive, but rather it intends to offer a manageable and sensible guide to protecting your loved one.

For more elaborate planning, please see the list of Resources at the end.

I'm sure you don't need reminding that it's important to be respectful toward caregivers. Their work is not easy. It's useful to assume that they want the best for your loved one and consider you an important part of the care team, unless or until you find out otherwise. Be sure to introduce yourself to each and every new healthcare worker. Let them know you are available to help in any way you can.

Recommendations to consider:

1. Make sure your loved one has an up-to-date Advance Directive. You can easily download the simple form applicable to your own state. The AD makes clear your loved one's wishes for care. It tells the medical team what treatment they do and do not want to be given, especially if they cannot make decisions for themselves and are suddenly faced with the end of their lives.

2. Make sure you obtain and keep copies of your loved one's medical records. Everyone has a right to their own medical record.[28] Each hospital has a medical records department from whom you can order copies.

3. Educate yourself about all the medical care they have received thus far as well as recommendations for further care and its reasons, taking into consideration the risks and benefits, i.e. what, if any, are the downsides of the treatment recommended? What are the odds that the treatment will be effective?

4. Make a list of all their medications, frequency, dosages, the illnesses for which they are prescribed and any potential side effects. Keep the list with you at all times and add to it as needed. THIS IS VERY IMPORTANT!! Had I not known that Steve had only 30,000 platelets at the time he was admitted to the ER (150,000 is low normal) and that heparin is a blood thinner, Steve likely would have died as a result of the doctor's negligence in not noticing his low platelet count. Upon review, the hospital even admitted that they had "counseled" that resident. Steve might not even have lived long enough to get a new liver if I'd not been there to block the shot.

5. Understand that you are in charge of your loved one's care, if they are not able to participate. In our case, Steve was not able to manage many of his own decisions; so it was up to me to make them for him.

6. Be aware that you have a right to know everything that's going on and a right to question everything.

7. Make sure that everyone who comes into the room washes their hands—including doctors, nurses, technicians and others!!

8. Regarding meds or IV's, make sure you know what has been prescribed and check each time with the nurse or doctor before they administer it. Make sure you read the label on the bottle or vial or bag. Mistakes can happen. In 2017 a nurse at Vanderbilt Hospital in Tennessee killed a patient by injecting her with the wrong drug. The woman's doctor had ordered the anti-anxiety medication Versed because she was claustrophobic and needed a CAT scan. The nurse became confused and instead of injecting her with Versed, she injected her with Vecuronium, a paralytic agent. The patient died two days later.[29]

A friend of my niece was hospitalized at an "excellent" hospital for his bone marrow transplant. Fortunately, his mother was staying with him. On one occasion a nurse arrived to give him a pill. His mother asked the nurse and was told what it was. Turns out that the drug was *the one* her son was allergic to! She stopped the nurse from giving it to her son. Who knows what might have happened if the mother had not stepped in?

9. If you are not able to stay 24/7 with your hospitalized loved one, please find another person or two to give you a break. Make sure they have all the information you have: your loved one's condition, including their medications, allergies, and treatment plans.

10. When in doubt, if a new procedure is suggested, make sure you get your questions answered before you give consent. Ask if it's an emergency; tell them to carefully

explain the risks/benefits to your loved one. Get a second opinion, if you can, just to make sure.

11. Call in a private duty nurse if needed and if you can afford it. I know that's a stretch for most people, but it is an alternative to consider. Contact your employer about the Family Medical Leave Act to find out how that might help you.

12. Know whom to contact in the hospital if you have a concern that's not being addressed by the doctors or nurses. Most hospitals have an ombudsman or a patient advocate on staff to assist when there are problems. Do not hesitate to call upon them. The assistance I received from the ombudsman at Steve's hospital was crucial to his eventually successful outcome.

13. Keep in mind that the intimate information you possess of your loved one is important to the success of their care. You deserve to be treated with respect and not dismissed as "difficult."

14. Do NOT let your loved one out of your sight, if you can help it. Go with them to their tests, i.e. MRI, CAT scans, surgery, etc. You will not be allowed in the same room for some of these procedures, but at least you will know where they are, and, just as importantly, they and the staff will know you are right outside. Make sure you give your cell phone number to one of the nurses and ask her to give you updates. And get the cell phone number of the hospital contact person.

I met a woman recently who told me about her experience with her husband at an "excellent" hospital where he was admitted for bladder surgery. Even as her husband was being prepped, a nurse came out to tell her that the anesthesiologist never showed up. This is NOT a good sign. They were going to cancel the operation unless they could get someone to fill in!

Half an hour later the woman received a phone call from another person in the hospital wanting to know where her husband was. *Where was he?!!* He had been transported to a different location within the huge medical complex, but apparently no one had documented his location in their computer system. And nobody bothered to call her.

They couldn't find him!

From there on, she said it got worse. A surgery that should have taken only two hours lasted seven, and no one was updating her each step of the way. The surgeon never stopped to talk to her, as promised. After that her husband developed sepsis, a life-threatening condition that occurs when the body's response to an infection damages its own organs and tissues. It's also known as septicemia or blood poisoning. Sepsis can lead to septic shock, organ failure, and even death if not diagnosed and treated early.

Her husband was also hospitalized for a month because of two bouts of cellulitis caused, she said, by dirty IVs. Cellulitis is a common bacterial skin infection that causes the skin to become warm, tender, and red, and may also cause blisters, chills, fever, and swollen lymph nodes.

In the end, her husband did survive but none of this should have happened.

She assumed, like many, that since her husband was in an "excellent" hospital, everything would be fine. In reviewing her story, it occurred to me that had she done a few simple things, she and her husband might have avoided much of this pain:

1. Stayed with her husband, wherever they took him. Obviously she couldn't follow him into the operating room, but it was important that she follow along as far as she could go and that the staff know she was just outside.

2. Made sure she had given her cell phone number to the nurse and asked to be updated. She could also have gotten the number of whom to call to get a status update, if one was not forthcoming within a reasonable amount of time.

3. Followed up with management about the "dirty IVs." As soon as she became aware of this problem, she should have filed a complaint to the Director of Quality Assurance at the hospital and later to the Joint Commission on Accreditation of Healthcare Organizations (JCAHO).[30]

Who would have dreamt that this could happen in an "excellent" hospital? What occurred was not her fault. Her husband was getting outrageously bad medical care which should NOT have happened, yet it did.

A few additional recommendations for everyone: Before you visit your own doctor, type up your reason for the visit in as few words as possible and ask them to read it. This serves two purposes: 1) to make sure your doctor knows exactly why you're there and 2) to save time. Ask them to add your note to your record. Keep a copy for yourself!

Whenever visiting a new physician, bring a brief summary of your medical history and medications. Doctors often have only

10-12 minutes, if that, to get up to speed. You want to save them as much time as possible. Every minute counts.

Do not hesitate to ask for a second opinion for any treatment, test or procedure, just to be sure you're making the right decision.

For more detailed information, please refer to the Resources section.

I hope these recommendations are useful. Some of you have your own horror stories. I would like to hear from you. Feel free to email them to me, in confidence at: medicalstories@yahoo.com. I may ask permission to use them in future articles or books.

My philosophy is this: Hope for the best, plan for the worst and, as the Girl Scouts say—"Be Prepared."

I wish the very best for you and your loved ones!

Please consult the Resources section for more information.

X. End Notes

1. Medical Errors Are No. 3 Cause Of U.S Deaths, Researchers Say
   www.npr.org/sections/health-shots/2016/05/03/476636183/death-certificates-
   undercount-toll-of-medical-errors
2. Report Highlights Public Health Impact of Serious Harms From Diagnostic
   Error in U.S." https://www.hopkinsmedicine.org/news/newsroom/news-
   releases/2023/07/report-highlights-public-health-impact-of-serious-harms-
   from-diagnostic-error-in-
   us#:~:text=Results%20of%20the%20new%20analysis,of%20the%20public%20h
   ealth%20problem
3. Medical Diagnosis Mistakes Kill or Disable 795,000 Americans Every Year
   https://www.everydayhealth.com/public-health/medical-diagnosis-mistakes-
   kill-or-disable-americans-every-year/
4. Deadly Pharmacy Errors Mount as Companies Push Quotas, Limit Staff: 'I Am
   a Danger to the Public. https://nypost.com/2023/09/05/deadly-pharmacy-
   errors-are-mounting-a-danger-to-the-public
5. California Pharmacies are Making Millions of Mistakes. They're failing to Keep
   That Secret. https://www.latimes.com/business/story/2023-09-05/california-
   pharmacies-prescription-errors-cvs-walgreens
6. How Chaos at Chain Pharmacies is Putting Patients at Risk
   https://www.nytimes.com/2020/01/31/health/pharmacists-medication-
   errors.html?searchResultPosition=4

7. Frustrated Pharmacists Could Go on Strike in Rare Protest. November 2023. https://www.nbcnews.com/business/business-news/pharmacy-strike-cvs-walgreens-rite-aid-worker-conditions-rcna121944

8. Doctors Aren't Burned Out from Overwork. We're Demoralized by Our Health System. www.nytimes.com/2023/02/05/opinion/doctors-universal-health-care-html

9. Medical Errors May Stem More From Physician Burnout than Unsafe Health Care Settings. https://med.stanford.edu/news/all-news/2018/07/medical-errors-may-stem-more-from-physician-burnout.html

10. Health Workforce Shortage Areas, May 4, 2024 https://data.hrsa.gov/topics/health-workforce/shortage-areas

11. AAMC Report Reinforces Mounting Physician Shortage, May 4, 202 https://www.aamc.org/news/press-releases/aamc-report-reinforces-mounting-physician-shortage#:~:text=According%20to%20new%20data%20published,both%20primary%20and%20specialty%20care

12. If I Betray These Words: Moral Injury in Medicine and Why It's So Hard for Clinicians to Put Patients First,; 2023, Wendy Dean, M.D.

13. Open Arms Veterans and Family Counseling Association https://www.openarms.gov.au/signs-symptoms/moral-injury#:~:text=Moral%20injury%20refers%20to%20the,associated%20with%20PTSD%20or%20depression

14. The Corporatization of Health Care has Changed the Practice of Medicine, Causing Many Physicians to Feel Alienated from Their Work. https://www.nytimes.com/2023/06/15/magazine/doctors-moral-crises.html

15. How Private Equity Firms Widen The Income Gap https://www.npr.org/2023/04/26/1172179099/how-private-equity-firms-widen-the-income-gap

16. Stop Private Equity from Driving Retailers into Bankruptcy, Destroying Jobs and Livelihoods. https://ourfinancialsecurity.org/2021/10/fact-sheet-stop-private-equity-from-driving-retailers-into-bankruptcy-destroying-jobs-and-livelihoods/

17. A Corporate Merger Cost America Ventilators https://www.nytimes.com/2020/04/12/opinion/ventilators-coronavirus.html

18. The U.S. Tried to build a New Fleet of Ventilators. The Mission Failed. https://www.nytimes.com/2020/03/29/business/coronavirus-us-ventilator-shortage.html

19. Assistant Secretary for Planning and Evaluation of Health Policy, February, 2022 www.aspe.hhs.gov

20. Hispanic/Latino - Office of Minority Health https://minorityhealth.hhs.gov

21. An Estimated 530,000 Families File for Bankruptcy Each Year Because of Medical Bills https://www.linkedin.com/pulse/medical-bankruptcy-crisis-affects-millions-americans-alex-koshykov-a9x7e/

22. Racial Bias in Pain Assessment and Treatment Recommendations, and False Beliefs About Biological Differences Between Blacks and Whites. Proceedings of the National Academy of Sciences of the United States, April 4, 2016 https://www.pnas.org/doi/10.1073/pnas.1516047113

23. AI Chatbot Answers on Health Questions Indicate Racial Bias. https://www.chiefhealthcareexecutive.com/view/ai-chatbot-answers-on-health-indicate-racial-bias

24. Nothing Protects Black Women From Dying in Pregnancy and Childbirth. https://www.propublica.org/article/nothing-protects-black-women-from-dying-in-pregnancy-and-childbirth

25. How Can We Solve the Black Maternal Health Crisis? https://publichealth.jhu.edu/2023/solving-the-black-maternal-health-crisis#:~:text=Black%20birthing%20people%20are%20also,birth%20and%20low%20birth%20weight.

26. Homicide During Pregnancy and the Postpartum Period in the United States, 2018–2019 https://www.journals.lww.com/greenjournal/Abstract/2021/11000/Homicide_During_Pregnancy_and_the_Postpartum.10.aspx

27. California Hospitals Ignored Bias Training Despite High Black Maternal Death Rate. https://www.kqed.org/news/11965919/california-hospitals-ignored-bias-training-despite-high-black-maternal-death-rate

28. HIPA (Health Insurance Portability and Accountability Act) Rules regarding patient's rights to obtain copies of their medical records as well as their right to privacy, 2022. https://www.hhs.gov/hipaa/for-individuals/guidance-materials-for-consumers/index.html

29. The Chilling Fate of the Nurse Who Accidentally Killed a Patient. April 26, 2022. https://slate.com/technology/2022/04/radonda-vaught-trial-vanderbilt-nurse-burnout.html

30. The public may contact the Joint Commission's Office of Quality Monitoring to report any concern or make a complaint about a health care facility that is accredited by the Joint Commission. https://www.jointcommission.org/resources/patient-safety-topics/report-a-patient-safety-concern-or-complaint

XI. Appendix

SB-464 California Dignity in Pregnancy and Childbirth Act

https://leginfo.legislature.ca.gov/faces/billNavClient.xhtml?bill_id=201920200SB464

Childbirth Act. (2019-2020)

Date Published: 10/08/2019 02:00 PM

BILL START

Senate Bill No. 464

CHAPTER 533

An act to amend Sections 1262.6 and 102875 of, and to add Article 4.6 (commencing with Section 123630) to Chapter 2 of Part 2 of Division 106 of, the Health and Safety Code, relating to maternal health.

[Approved by Governor October 07, 2019. Filed with Secretary of State October 07, 2019.]

LEGISLATIVE COUNSEL'S DIGEST

SB 464, Mitchell. California Dignity in Pregnancy and Childbirth Act.

(1) Existing law requires the State Department of Public Health to maintain a program of maternal and child health, which may include, among other things, facilitating services directed toward reducing infant mortality and improving the health of mothers and children. Existing law requires the Office of Health Equity within the department to serve as a resource for ensuring that programs collect and keep data and information regarding ethnic and racial health statistics, and strategies and programs that address multicultural health issues, including, but not limited to, infant and maternal mortality.

This bill would make legislative findings relating to implicit bias and racial disparities in maternal mortality rates. The bill would require a hospital that provides perinatal care, and an alternative birth center or a primary clinic that provides services as an alternative birth center, to implement an evidence-based implicit bias program, as specified, for all health care providers involved in perinatal care of patients within those facilities. The bill would require the health care provider to complete initial basic training through the program and a refresher course every 2 years thereafter, or on a more frequent basis if deemed necessary by the facility. The bill would require the facility to provide a certificate of training completion upon request, to accept certificates of completion from other facilities, and to offer training to physicians not directly employed by the facility.

The bill would require the department to track and publish data on pregnancy-related death and severe maternal morbidity, as specified.

(2) Existing law requires that each death be registered with the local registrar of births and deaths in the district in which the death was officially pronounced or the body was found. Existing law sets forth the persons responsible for completing the certificate of death and requires certain medical and health content on the certificate, including information indicating whether the decedent was pregnant at the time of death or within the year prior to the death, if known. Certain violations of these requirements are a crime.

This bill would require the certificate to indicate additional information regarding the pregnancy status of the decedent, as specified. By changing the definition of existing crimes, the bill would impose a state-mandated local program.

(3) Existing law requires hospitals to provide specified information regarding patient's rights to each patient upon admission or as soon thereafter as reasonably practical, including, among other things, information about the right to be informed of continuing health care requirements following discharge from the hospital. Existing law makes violations of these requirements a crime.

This bill would require the hospital to additionally provide patients with information on the patient's right to be free of discrimination on the basis of race, color, religion, ancestry, national origin, disability, medical condition, genetic information, marital status, sex, gender, gender identity, gender expression, sexual orientation, citizenship, primary language, or immigration status. The bill would additionally require the hospital to provide patients with information on how to file a complaint with specified state entities. By expanding the scope of a crime, this bill would impose a state-mandated local program.

(4) The California Constitution requires the state to reimburse local agencies and school districts for certain costs mandated by the state. Statutory provisions establish procedures for making that reimbursement.

This bill would provide that no reimbursement is required by this act for a specified reason.

BILL TEXT

THE PEOPLE OF THE STATE OF CALIFORNIA DO ENACT AS FOLLOWS:

SECTION 1.

Section 1262.6 of the Health and Safety Code is amended to read:

1262.6.

(a) Each hospital shall provide each patient, upon admission or as soon thereafter as reasonably practical, written information regarding the patient's right to the following:

(1) To be informed of continuing health care requirements following discharge from the hospital.

(2) To be informed that, if the patient so authorizes, that a friend or family member may be provided information about the patient's continuing health care requirements following discharge from the hospital.

(3) Participate actively in decisions regarding medical care. To the extent permitted by law, participation shall include the right to refuse treatment.

(4) Appropriate pain assessment and treatment consistent with Sections 124960 and 124961.

(5) To be free of discrimination on the basis of race, color, religion, ancestry, national origin, disability, medical condition, genetic information, marital status, sex, gender, gender identity, gender expression, sexual orientation, citizenship, primary

language, or immigration status as set forth in Section 51 of the Civil Code.

(6) Information on how to file a complaint with the following:

(A) The State Department of Public Health, in accordance with Section 1288.4.

(B) The Department of Fair Employment and Housing.

(C) The Medical Board of California.

(b) A hospital may include the information required by this section with other notices to the patient regarding patient rights. If a hospital chooses to include this information along with existing notices to the patient regarding patient rights, any newly required information shall be provided when the hospital exhausts its existing inventory of written materials and prints new written materials.

SEC. 2.

Section 102875 of the Health and Safety Code is amended to read:

102875.

The certificate of death shall be divided into two sections.

(a) The first section shall contain those items necessary to establish the fact of the death, including all of the following and those other items as the State Registrar may designate:

(1) (A) Personal data of decedent including full name, sex, color or race, marital status, name of spouse, date of birth and age at death, birthplace, usual residence, occupation and industry or business, and whether the decedent was ever in the Armed Forces of the United States.

(B) A person completing the certificate shall record the decedent's sex to reflect the decedent's gender identity. The decedent's gender identity shall be reported by the informant, unless the person completing the certificate is presented with a birth certificate, a driver's license, a social security record, a court order approving a name or gender change, a passport, an advanced health care directive, or proof of clinical treatment for gender transition, in which case the person completing the certificate shall record the decedent's sex as that which corresponds to the decedent's gender identity as indicated in that document. If none of these documents are presented and the person with the right, or a majority of persons who have equal rights, to control the disposition of the remains pursuant to Section 7100 is in disagreement with the gender identity reported by the informant, the gender identity of the decedent recorded on the death certificate shall be as reported by that person or majority of persons.

(C) If a document specified in subparagraph (B) is not presented and a majority of persons who have equal rights to control the disposition of the remains pursuant to Section 7100 do not agree with the gender identity of the decedent as reported by the informant, any one of those persons may file a petition, in the superior court in the county in which the decedent resided at the time of the decedent's death, or in which the remains are located, naming as a party to the action those persons who otherwise have equal rights to control the disposition and seeking an order of the court determining, as appropriate, who among those parties shall determine the gender identity of the decedent.

(D) A person completing the death certificate in compliance with subparagraph (B) is not liable for any damages or costs arising from claims related to the sex of the decedent as entered on the certificate of death.

(E) A person completing the death certificate shall comply with the data and certification requirements described in Section

102800 by using the information available to the person prior to the deadlines for completion specified in that section.

(2) Date of death, including month, day, and year.

(3) Place of death.

(4) Full name of father and birthplace of father, and full maiden name of mother and birthplace of mother.

(5) Informant.

(6) Disposition of body information, including signature and license number of embalmer, if the body is embalmed, or name of embalmer if affixed by attorney-in-fact; name of funeral director, or person acting as such; and date and place of interment or removal. Notwithstanding any other law, an electronic signature substitute, or some other indicator of authenticity, approved by the State Registrar may be used in lieu of the actual signature of the embalmer.

(7) Certification and signature of attending physician and surgeon or certification and signature of coroner when required to act by law. Notwithstanding any other law, the person completing the portion of the certificate setting forth the cause of death may attest to its accuracy by use of an electronic signature substitute, or some other indicator of authenticity, approved by the State Registrar in lieu of a signature.

(8) Date accepted for registration and signature of local registrar. Notwithstanding any other law, the local registrar may elect to use an electronic signature substitute, or some other indicator of authenticity, approved by the State Registrar in lieu of a signature.

(b) The second section shall contain those items relating to medical and health data, including all of the following and other items as the State Registrar may designate:

(1) Disease or conditions leading directly to death and antecedent causes.

(2) Operations and major findings thereof.

(3) Accident and injury information.

(4) Information indicating whether the decedent was pregnant at the time of death, or within a year prior to the death, if known, as determined by observation, autopsy, or review of the medical record. The electronic death registration system shall capture additional information regarding the pregnancy status of the decedent consistent with the data elements on the U.S. Standard Certificate of Death. This paragraph shall not be interpreted to require the performance of a pregnancy test on a decedent, or to require a review of medical records in order to determine pregnancy.

SEC. 3.

Article 4.6 (commencing with Section 123630) is added to Chapter 2 of Part 2 of Division 106 of the Health and Safety Code, to read:

Article 4.6. California Dignity in Pregnancy and Childbirth Act

123630.

This article shall be known, and may be cited, as the California Dignity in Pregnancy and Childbirth Act.

123630.1.

The Legislature hereby finds and declares all of the following:

(a) Every person should be entitled to dignity and respect during and after pregnancy and childbirth. Patients should receive the best care possible regardless of their race, gender, age, class, sexual orientation, gender identity, disability, language proficiency, nationality, immigration status, gender expression, or religion.

(b) The United States has the highest maternal mortality rate in the developed world. About 700 women die each year from childbirth, and another 50,000 suffer from severe complications. In California, since 2006, the rate of maternal death has decreased 55 percent, in contrast to the steady increase in the United States as a whole.

(c) However, for women of color, particularly Black women, the maternal mortality rate remains three to four times higher than White women. Black women make up 5 percent of the pregnancy cohort in California, but 21 percent of the pregnancy-related deaths.

(d) Forty-one percent of all pregnancy-related deaths had a good to strong chance of preventability. California has a responsibility to decrease the number of preventable pregnancy-related deaths.

(e) Pregnancy-related deaths among Black women are also more likely to be miscoded. Thirty-five percent of pregnancy-related deaths among Black women in California were miscoded, misidentifying pregnancy-related deaths as other deaths.

(f) Access to prenatal care, socioeconomic status, and general physical health do not fully explain the disparity seen in Black women's maternal mortality and morbidity rates. There is a growing body of evidence that Black women are often treated unfairly and unequally in the health care system.

(g) Implicit bias is a key cause that drives health disparities in communities of color. At present, health care providers in California are not required to undergo any implicit bias testing or training. Nor does there exist any system to track the number of incidents where implicit prejudice and implicit stereotypes have led to negative birth and maternal health outcomes.

(h) It is the intent of the Legislature to reduce the effects of implicit bias in pregnancy, childbirth, and postnatal care so that all people are treated with dignity and respect by their health care providers.

123630.2.

For the purposes of this article, the following terms have the following meanings:

(a) "Pregnancy-related death" is the death of a person while pregnant or within 365 days of the end of a pregnancy, irrespective of the duration or site of the pregnancy, from any cause related to, or aggravated by, the pregnancy or its management, but not from accidental or incidental causes.

(b) "Implicit bias" is a bias in judgment or behavior that results from subtle cognitive processes, including implicit prejudice and implicit stereotypes that often operate at a level below conscious awareness and without intentional control.

(c) "Implicit prejudice" is prejudicial negative feelings or beliefs about a group that a person holds without being aware of them.

(d) "Implicit stereotypes" are the unconscious attributions of particular qualities to a member of a certain social group. Implicit stereotypes are influenced by experience and are based on learned associations between various qualities and social categories, including race or gender.

(e) "Perinatal care" is the provision of care during pregnancy, labor, delivery, and postpartum and neonatal periods.

123630.3.

(a) A hospital as defined in subdivision (a) or (f) of Section 1250 that provides perinatal care, and an alternative birth center or primary care clinic subject to Section 1204.3, shall implement an evidence-based implicit bias program for all health care providers involved in the perinatal care of patients within those facilities.

(b) An implicit bias program implemented pursuant to subdivision (a) shall include all of the following:

(1) Identification of previous or current unconscious biases and misinformation.

(2) Identification of personal, interpersonal, institutional, structural, and cultural barriers to inclusion.

(3) Corrective measures to decrease implicit bias at the interpersonal and institutional levels, including ongoing policies and practices for that purpose.

(4) Information on the effects, including, but not limited to, ongoing personal effects, of historical and contemporary exclusion and oppression of minority communities.

(5) Information about cultural identity across racial or ethnic groups.

(6) Information about communicating more effectively across identities, including racial, ethnic, religious, and gender identities.

(7) Discussion on power dynamics and organizational decisionmaking.

(8) Discussion on health inequities within the perinatal care field, including information on how implicit bias impacts maternal and infant health outcomes.

(9) Perspectives of diverse, local constituency groups and experts on particular racial, identity, cultural, and provider-community relations issues in the community.

(10) Information on reproductive justice.

(c) (1) A health care provider described in subdivision (a) shall complete initial basic training through the implicit bias program based on the components described in subdivision (b).

(2) Upon completion of the initial basic training, a health care provider shall complete a refresher course under the implicit bias program every two years thereafter, or on a more frequent basis if deemed necessary by the facility, in order to keep current with changing racial, identity, and cultural trends and best practices in decreasing interpersonal and institutional implicit bias.

(d) A facility described in subdivision (a) shall provide a certificate of training completion to another facility or a training attendee upon request. A facility may accept a certificate of completion from another facility described in subdivision (a) to satisfy the training requirement described in subdivision (c) from a health care provider who works in more than one facility.

(e) Notwithstanding subdivisions (a) to (d), inclusive, if a physician involved in the perinatal care of patients is not directly employed by a facility, the facility shall offer the training to the physician.

123630.4.

(a) The State Department of Public Health shall track data on severe maternal morbidity, including, but not limited to, all of the following health conditions:

(1) Obstetric hemorrhage.

(2) Hypertension.

(3) Preeclampsia and eclampsia.

(4) Venous thromboembolism.

(5) Sepsis.

(6) Cerebrovascular accident.

(7) Amniotic fluid embolism.

(b) The data on severe maternal morbidity collected pursuant to subdivision (a) shall be published at least once every three years, after all of the following have occurred:

(1) The data has been aggregated by state regions, as defined by the State Department of Public Health, to ensure data reflects how regionalized care systems are or should be collaborating to improve maternal health outcomes, or other smaller regional sorting based on standard statistical methods for accurate dissemination of public health data without risking a confidentiality or other disclosure breach.

(2) The data has been disaggregated by racial and ethnic identity.

(c) The State Department of Public Health shall track data on pregnancy-related deaths, including, but not limited to, all of the conditions listed in subdivision (a), indirect obstetric deaths, and other maternal disorders predominantly related to pregnancy and complications predominantly related to the puerperium.

(d) The data on pregnancy-related deaths collected pursuant to subdivisions (a) and (c) shall be published, at least once every three years, after all of the following have occurred:

(1) The data has been aggregated by state regions, as defined by the State Department of Public Health, to ensure data reflects how regionalized care systems are or should be collaborating to improve maternal health outcomes, or other smaller regional sorting based on standard statistical methods for accurate dissemination of public health data without risking a confidentiality or other disclosure breach.

(2) The data has been disaggregated by racial and ethnic identity.

SEC. 4.

No reimbursement is required by this act pursuant to Section 6 of Article XIII B of the California Constitution because the only costs that may be incurred by a local agency or school district will be incurred because this act creates a new crime or infraction, eliminates a crime or infraction, or changes the penalty for a crime or infraction, within the meaning of Section 17556 of the Government Code, or changes the definition of a crime within the meaning of Section 6 of Article XIII B of the California Constitution.

RESOURCES

Rana Awdish, M.D. (2017) *In Shock: My Journey From Death to Recovery and the Redemptive Power of Hope,* St. Martin's Press.

Theresa Brown, R.N. (2022) *Healing: When a Nurse Becomes a Patient.* Algonquin.

Wendy Dean, M.D. (2023) *If I Betray These Words: Moral Injury in Medicine And Why It's So Hard for Clinicians to Put Patients First.* Steerforth Press.

Robert Fox, J.D., and Chris Landon, M.D. (2020) *Avoiding Medical Errors: One Hundred Rules to Help You Survive Mistakes by Doctors and Hospitals,* Rowman & Littlefield.

Sana Goldberg, R.N. (2017) *How to Be a Patient: The Essential Guide to Navigating the World of Modern Medicine,* Gale.

Sorrell King (2009) *Josie's Story: A Mother's Inspiring Crusade to Make Medical Care Safe,* Atlantic Monthly Press.

Leapfrog Hospital Safety Grade. This is a public service provided by The Leapfrog Group, an independent nonprofit organization committed to driving quality. You can look up information about any hospital in the country. https://www.hospitalsafetygrade.org

Marty Makary, M.D. (2019) *The Price We Pay: What Broke American Health Care — and How to Fix It,* Bloomsbury.

Marty Makary, M.D., (2012) *Unaccountable: What Hospitals Won't Tell You and How Transparency Can Revolutionize Health Care,* Bloomsbury.

Gretchen Morgenson and Joshua Rosner (2023*) These are the Plunderers: How Private Equity Runs—and—Wrecks America,* Simon and Schuster.

Danielle Ofri, M.D. (2020) *When We Do Harm: A Doctor Confronts Medical Error,* Beacon Press.

Danielle Ofri, M.D. (2017) *What Patients Say, What* Doctors Hear, Beacon Press.

Elisabeth Rosenthal, M.D. (2017) *An American Sickness: How Healthcare Became Big Business and How You Can Take it Back,* Penguin Press.

Linda Villarosa, (2022) *Under the Skin: The Hidden Toll of Racism on American Lives and On the Health of Our Nation,* Double Day.

Harriet Washington (2008) *Medical Apartheid: The Dark History of Medical Experimentation on Black Americans from Colonial Times to the Present,* Penguin Random House.

ACKNOWLEDGMENTS

I wish to begin by thanking the authors of all the books I have ever read, beginning with the authors of *Fun with Dick and Jane*. Thank you, thank you, thank you for cracking open my mind.

Next, a special shout out to Mrs. Reeser, my first grade teacher, who, with her love of phonics, made sure all 15 of us could read by the end of the year.

Another round of applause goes to all the librarians who will fight to the death anyone who seeks to desecrate those hallowed stacks. Woe to anyone who intends on hijacking civilization by banning books. They don't know with whom they are dealing!

Gratitude of the oceanic kind to all the people who read my early drafts and who are still my friends:

Cheryl Thompson, the best sis-in-law a girl could have. Jay Thompson, the best cousin a girl could have. Jill Kneeter, the best Speech Director I ever hired; she always laughs at my jokes. Ann Allen, world's best cat advocate and big fan of my political satire.

Dr. Deborah Joy, whose kindness and smarts have buoyed me, lo these many years. Dr. Bob Nozik and Marsha Colby, Taylor Teegarden, Sue Bartlett, Colleen Rae and Jeff Woodruff for our friendship of many many years. Deborah and David Erickson for cheering me on. We miss you, Deborah.

Dr. Benedicte Dahlerup, who understands the problem of medical errors and appreciated my desire to tell people about them.

And, to my dear departed brilliant writer friend, Grant Flint, who cheered me on from the moment I sat down at my IBM Selectric and who lived long enough to see many of my words (now word processed) find publication. To his children Scott and Angie Flint and grandchildren, Jared Flint and Katrina Unpingco who carry on Grant's tradition of kindness and generosity.

MY EDITORS

Jonathan Odell, without whose encouragement I would never have finished the book. Probably wouldn't even have started. If you want to indulge in a banquet of fine Southern fried stories, check out Jon's novels.

Lingsie Jensen, fellow Scandie, whose eagle eye saved me from many an embarrassing mistake. To Kurt Jensen, her husband and also dear friend, who cheered me on and baked me the best buns I've ever eaten.

Guy Biederman, the finest teacher, editor, cat lover and friend a writer could have.

Carol Clurman, who encouraged me to add more personal stories.

To Elizabeth Fishel, who kindly referred me to Carol when she was overwhelmed with her other projects.

Dr. Carolyn Ingram, writer, poet, psychologist and coach. There's no one better at understanding and guiding others to success.

Eve Nilson, another fellow Scandie and bookseller extraordinaire. Check out her offerings at "Eve's Book Garden" at Abebooks.com.

Brooke Warner, champion of memoirists everywhere, whose advice I very much appreciated. It's been a pleasure these past 15 years, watching her grow from editor to coach to Publisher of She Writes Press and author. She is making a profound impact on the publishing industry.

Additional gratitude to Daidre West for her support throughout Steve's horror show and to Jan Schrock, who trekked more than three thousand miles to be with her dear brother during the early days of his recovery. Wish she could be here to read the book.

A special thanks to Eva Natiello, who shows by example and expert instruction how an independent author can succeed. And, she's fun!

Many thanks to Dr. Chris Nizer, world's best upper cervical chiropractor, who has kept my body and soul together for the past seven years.

Special thanks to Steve's son, Landon West, who saved my life by arriving when he did. There are not enough words to convey my gratitude for all his support. Thanks, Dude!

Much gratitude to Nadine Reinhardt, my book designer. I've never met anyone as dedicated to customer happiness as is Nadine. And, she was fun to work with!

And, of course, the man without whom this book would never have been written and who has edited it more times than we can count: Steve West. Happy you made it home alive, Sweetheart! Aren't you glad I'm finally done?

ABOUT THE AUTHOR

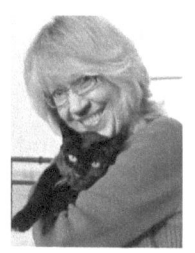 Rosie Sorenson, MA, MFT, is a former healthcare administrator and psychotherapist.

Rosie's work has appeared in the *Literary Medical Messenger*, the *Los Angeles Times, Mobius,* the *Chicago Tribune,* the San Francisco Chronicle, the Pittsburgh Tribune-Review, the University of Iowa Daily Palette and others.

Her essays appear in popular anthologies, including the *Magic of Memoir: Inspiration for the Writing Journey.*

In addition, she has been writing political satire for the *Progressive Populist* for the past six years. Prior to that she wrote a humor column for the *Foolish Times* for ten years.

Awards

Lee Child, Judge for the Black Spring Prize for Best Openings to a Crime Book, included Rosie's entry in the top 100—*Crime Bits: 100 Opening Gambits for Great Thrillers.*

The 2023 San Francisco Writers' Conference 2023 Writing Contest: Finalist for the Introduction to her new memoir: *If*

You'd Only Listen: A Medical Memoir of Gaslighting, Grit and Grace, published in their anthology, *What We've Believed.*

The Joyce Turley Scholarship from the 2020 San Francisco Writers Conference for an essay.

The Listener Favorite Award from the popular San Francisco NPR affiliate in its "Perspectives" series.

Winner in the essay competition from the Writers College, UK and NZ.

Honorable Mention in the Erma Bombeck Writing Contest.

Muse Medallion Award from the Cat Writer's Association for *They Had Me at Meow: Tails of Love from the Homeless Cats of Buster Hollow.*

Rosie lives with her Sweetheart Steve in Northern California and their beloved cat, Billy.

For more information, please visit her website: www.RosieSorenson.com

Note to Reader

Thank you for reading my book. I hope it was enjoyable as well as helpful. If you liked it, would you please write a brief review on Amazon? No need for a long dissertation, but a few words would be appreciated. As you might know, authors live and die by Amazon reviews! You can also write directly to me at: RosieSorenson29@yahoo.com.

Thank you very much.

www.ingramcontent.com/pod-product-compliance
Lightning Source LLC
Chambersburg PA
CBHW030909120626
46554CB00001B/66